Stories in Chronic Illness and Disability:
Reflection, Inquiry, Action

Stories in Chronic Illness and Disability:
Reflection, Inquiry, Action

Edited by Esther Chang and Amanda Johnson

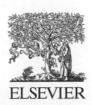

ELSEVIER

ELSEVIER

Elsevier Australia. ACN 001 002 357
(a division of Reed International Books Australia Pty Ltd)
Tower 1, 475 Victoria Avenue, Chatswood, NSW 2067

ISBN: 978-0-7295-4404-7

National Library of Australia Cataloguing-in-Publication Data

 A catalogue record for this book is available from the National Library of Australia

Head of Content Strategy: Natalie Hunt
Content Project Manager: Shubham Dixit
Edited by Jo Crichton
Proofread by Tim Learner
Cover by Gopalakrishnan Venkatraman
Typeset by Aptara
Printed in China by 1010 Printing International Ltd

Last digit is the print number: 9 8 7 6 5 4 3 2 1

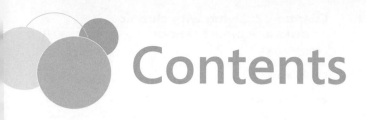

Contents

Contents

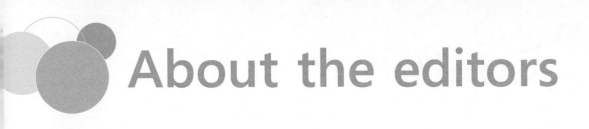

About the editors

Esther Chang, RN, CM, DNE, BAppSc(AdvNurs), MEdAdmin, PhD, FRCNA

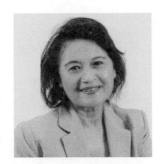

Professor Esther Chang is an Emeritus Professor at the Western Sydney University. She is a Registered Nurse and a Midwife. She has worked in academia since 1986 with three tertiary institutions. She has held roles as a Clinical Nurse Educator, Head of School, Dean of the Faculty of Health, Acting Pro Vice-Chancellor Academic, Director of International and Business, Director of Research and Director of Higher Degree Research. Professor Chang's research for over 25 years has been in aged care, with an emphasis on models of care for people with dementia and palliation. She has co-edited over 20 books to assist students in tertiary institutions, new registered nurses, and clinicians to improve health care and provide guidance for future generations of nurses and midwives.

Amanda Johnson, RN, DipT(Nurs), MSc(HEd), PhD

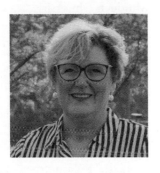

Professor Amanda Johnson is a Professor of Nursing at the University of Newcastle where she holds the role of Head of School, Dean of Nursing and Midwifery and Campus Lead for the Central Coast Clinical School. She is a Registered Nurse, having worked in academia since 1992 with three tertiary institutions holding senior management positions. Professor Johnson has been the recipient of a Vice Chancellors Excellence in Teaching Award (Highly Commended) for her work in chronic illness and disability having established the subject and co-edited a textbook, now in its 4th edition to support student's learning and the delivery of optimal care. Professor Johnson has a commitment to excellence in care for vulnerable people and continues to research in aged care and palliation using this knowledge to inform undergraduate nursing curricula and professional placement experiences culminating in the preparation of graduates for future practice.

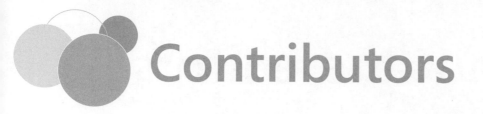

Contributors

Sharon Andrews
RN, BN(Hons), PhD
Associate Professor, School of Nursing
University of Tasmania
Rozelle, NSW, Australia

Robert Batterbee
BSc(Hons), PGDip(CBT), Credentialed Mental
Health Nurse, PhD Candidate
Lecturer, Generalist and Mental Health Nursing
College of Science, Health, Engineering and
Education
Murdoch University
WA, Australia

Ginger Chu
PhD
Doctor, School of Nursing and Midwifery
University of Newcastle
Callaghan, NSW, Australia

Ritin Fernandez
PhD
Professor, School of Nursing and Midwifery
University of Newcastle
NSW, Australia

Jane Frost
RN, BSc(Hons), MSCNP, DNP, GCTE, PFHEA
Professor, School of Nursing and Midwifery
Western Sydney University
NSW, Australia;
Adjunct Professor, Faculty of Health
University of Canberra
ACT, Australia;
Adjunct Associate Professor, Nursing and
Midwifery
Edith Cowan University
WA, Australia

Eleanor Horton
PhD, MHlthSc (Nsg), BHlthSc(Nsg), ADN, RN
Doctor
Queensland, Australia

Sara Karacsony
PhD
Doctor, School of Nursing, College of Health and
Medicine
University of Tasmania
NSW, Australia

Cannas Kwok
PhD, MPH, MEd, BHS(Nursing)
Associate Professor, Faculty of Science and Health
Charles Sturt University
Bathurst, NSW, Australia

Michelle Stubbs
PhD Nursing, Master of Nursing, Graduate
Diploma in Nursing, Graduate Certificate in
Anaesthetics and Recovery Room Nursing,
Bachelor of Nursing
Associate Professor, School of Nursing and
Midwifery
College of Health, Medicine and Wellbeing
University of Newcastle
NSW, Australia

Nathan J. Wilson
PhD, Grad Cert Sc(Applied Statistics), MSc,
BSocSc, Dip.HealthSc (Nursing)
Professor, School of Nursing and Midwifery
Western Sydney University
NSW, Australia

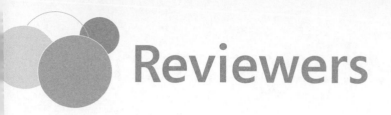

Reviewers

Kit Doudney
PhD
Senior Lecturer, Department of Nursing
University of Otago Christchurch
Christchurch, New Zealand

David Foley
PhD, MNS, CEN, RN, BSc
Adelaide Nursing School
Adelaide Health & Medical Sciences Building
University of Adelaide
SA, Australia

Colleen Van Lochem
RN, BN, MN, PG Cert Critical Care, MACN
Lecturer & Course Coordinator
Faculty of Medicine, Nursing and Midwifery and
    Health Sciences
National School of Nursing & Midwifery
University of Notre Dame
WA, Australia

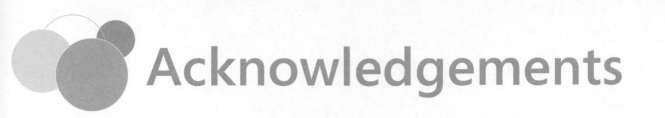

Acknowledgements

Acknowledgements and gratitude go to all the women, men and clinicians who contributed their time and freely told their stories. These contributions will enhance the development, knowledge and professionalism of health professionals and carers providing quality of care to people living with chronic illness and disability.

Aaron

Jamie

Grant

Bonnie

Jacqueline

Rebecca

Peter

Clare

Holly

Karen

Nell

Bronwen

Melissa

Eleanor

Zoe

Karen

Lois

Nicholas

Sharon

Heather

Dave

Carla

Sarah

Thida

Rebecca

Ruth

Jane

Linda

Joey

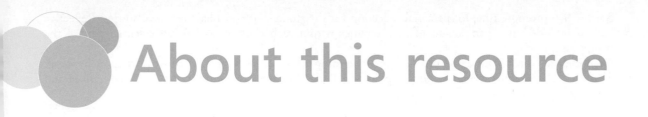

About this resource

Overview

This resource has been developed for tertiary nursing students, students in the TAFE sector, newly registered nurses and other health professionals who share our commitment to providing quality of care to people living with chronic illness and disability.

This resource is also based on the stories of people living with chronic illness and disability. It discusses the issues and challenges for health professionals and carers providing quality of care to people living with chronic illness and disability.

The aim of this book is to give students a better understanding of the lived experiences of people with chronic illness and disability. Learners will find viewpoints that are challenging and sometimes disconcerting, but at the same time motivating and thought provoking. Research has shed much light on the issues associated with chronic illness and disability, and has uncovered knowledge, including strategies that can be useful in negotiating the process of partnership with empathy.

Using the resource

Our intention was to involve clinicians, academics and people with chronic illness and disability and their carers, in producing a resource that is scholarly, accessible, reality-based and practical.

By reading the book, watching the videos, critically reflecting on the issues and posing possible answers, learners will be able to gain a comprehensive view of the issues, challenges and opportunities that lie ahead for them.

This resource can be also used as a tool for teaching and learning, critical reflection, inquiry and action, guiding the teacher and student through each chapter and at the same time allowing the learner to examine their beliefs and assumptions that have influenced their practice.

Research articles and chapters in books have also been selected for your reading and consideration as you progress through this comprehensive resource book. Each section has been provided to enable you to reflect on what you have learned in relation to people with health needs by reviewing the Registered Nurse Standards: https://www.nursingmidwiferyboard.gov.au

Structure of the resource

There are several constructs, key elements and questions that have guided authors within each chapter.

The stories

Storytelling brings lived experiences to life and helps the learner to remember key facts, as stories are easy to remember. Organisational psychologist Peg Neuhauser (1993) found that learners remembered more accurately and for far longer by storytelling. She believes that telling stories is one of the most powerful means that leaders and, in this case, teachers can influence, teach, inspire and motivate their learners.

Telling stories forges connections among people by bringing in history, culture and values that unite people and, in this case, your patients or clients, their families, or carers. It also allows you to have a better understanding of the needs and person-centred care for the individual.

Stories also promote time for personal reflection for the student to consider their own stories. Reflective practice is included as a component of the activities within each chapter, as it is an essential part of the learning process.

Each chapter focuses on a specific key understanding which is identified within the chapter heading. Within each chapter are several headings including Reflection, Inquiry and Action, with references and further reading lists at the end of the book.

Reflection

The learner is asked to think about what they have listened to and make some personal judgement on this information. There are several questions that will help with this process and guide key learnings. This section is useful for learners at all levels.

Inquiry

This section has been written to help the learner consider what else they need to know as well as identify any gaps in the knowledge presented that needs to be considered, along with potential solutions.

Action

This is divided into three questions: 1, 2 and 3.

Within this section, the learner is invited to apply their knowledge and understanding to not only their personal practice but also to the organisational and political frameworks in which their practice is embedded.

This section has been organised within a stepping-up framework:

1. Generally, asks the learner to apply their knowledge within the boundaries of their own personal practice.
2. Starts to introduce the notions of action within an organsational structure.
3. Generally, asks for the knowledge gained to be applied within the greater political framework.

It should be noted that it:
1. will be better focused for the certificate level learner
2. will be more for the undergraduate learner
3. is intended to stimulate inquiry for the postgraduate learner.

This provides all learners with the opportunity to consolidate their foundational understandings of the data presented before moving on to the more complex concepts identified at the next level. Learners can advance to the next area if they wish and consider the learnings from these notions.

Further reading

Mather, C., & Almond, H. C. (2024). Critically reflective practice for the graduate. In E. Chang, & D. Hatcher (Eds.), *Transitions in nursing: Preparing for professional practice* (6th ed.). Elsevier.

Neuhauser, P. C. (1993). *Corporate legends and lore: The power of storytelling as a management tool.* McGraw-Hill.

Rolfe, G., & Freshwater, D. (2020). *Critical reflection in practice: Generating knowledge for care.* Bloomsbury Publishing.

White, J. (2024). Becoming a competent, confident, professional registered nurse. In E. Chang, & D. Hatcher (Eds.), *Transitions in nursing: Preparing for professional practice* (6th ed.). Elsevier.

CHAPTER 1

Introduction: Perspectives on chronic illness and disability

Esther Chang, Amanda Johnson

INTRODUCTION

This introductory chapter will help you understand how people with chronic illness and disability continue to be a high priority of care globally for all governments. Throughout this text the form of expression *chronic disease*, *condition* and/or *illness* are used interchangeably. Specifically using chronic illness refers to the experience a person has of a chronic disease or long-term condition. Chronic illness may be experienced either independently or co-related to disability. The stories in this book come from a group of people who were willing to share their stories with you. The stories also come from carers and health professionals who provided care for them.

Before you begin

Think about your own views of disability in relation to chronic illness.

How do your perceptions reflect who you are and what experiences you have been through? It is important for nurses to examine their own beliefs and opinions that influence their behaviour when they care for people with chronic illness and disability. Our beliefs shape the way we think and influence our belief system. For the majority, our upbringing plays an important part in shaping how we perceive the world. As a nurse working with and caring for people with chronic illness and complex needs, you will also encounter spirituality flowing through people's lives and the experiences of illness, disability, suffering and wellbeing.

Questioning your beliefs can lead to change, but it can lead to reaffirming what you already believe about yourself. It also validates what is true for you. It influences the way you connect with people, and how you empathise with them as you communicate with them.

The following are some questions that would be helpful to ask yourself.

- What factors influence my beliefs and values?
- What are belief systems?
- How do thoughts, words and beliefs shape my actions?

- How does my belief system impact on my decisions?
- Why is it important not to make assumptions about people?
- What impact do beliefs, values and behaviour have on practice in my role as a nurse?

  These are the same questions that every practising nurse should ask themselves.

Chronic illness

In this text and in the textbook *Living with chronic illness and disability: Principles for nursing practice* (Chang & Johnson, 2022), the editors have selected chronic illness as a form of expression. This was chosen because it emphasises the human experience of the disease, as experienced by the person. Larson (2016) describes chronic illness as 'the lived experience of the individual and family diagnosed with a chronic disease' (pp. 5–6). It is important that healthcare professionals address the individual's and family's needs holistically (Larson, 2019).

Disability

Globally, The International Classification of Functioning, Disability and Health (2001) (Fifty-Fourth World Health Assembly, 2001) defines a person as being disabled when a level of difficulty is experienced in one or more of the following interconnecting areas.

- Impairment. A person with an impairment experiences issues related to body function or alteration to body structure (World Health Organization, 2011).
- Limitations. In this area, the person faces challenges in conducting everyday activities (WHO, 2011).
- Participation restrictions. In this area, an individual faces problems in any area of their life, not just health related (WHO 2011).

In relation to chronic disease, a person may experience disability independent of the disease state; for example, a person who has arthritis but develops cardiovascular disease; or disability may be a consequence of the disease.

The following are questions that would be helpful to consider.

- What assumptions do you hold about people with chronic illness and disability?
- How has your belief system affected how you do things for others?
- Have you, or any family members, suffered with chronic illness?
- Have you, or any family members, suffered with a disability?
- Has your own experience changed because of the experience?
- Why was it changed?

The global perspective of chronic disease

Now more than ever, there is a need to globally prevent and control the rise of chronic disease. The world and individual countries, whether low, middle or high income, can no longer sustain the human, social, economic and health impacts of chronic disease either now or in the future. It is the poor and vulnerable populations who are at risk (WHO, 2014). Furthermore, chronic conditions are an ongoing cause of substantial ill health, disability and premature death, making them an important global, national and individual health concern (Australian Institute of Health and Welfare, 2020). WHO reports that, by 2030, it is projected that chronic disease will account for 82% (55 million) of all deaths worldwide, which is an increase of 17 million since 2012 (WHO, 2013).

Chronic disease is a long-lasting condition with persistent impact on the individual from either the disease itself, the related treatments and/or the presence of two or more chronic conditions at the same time (AIHW, 2021), referred to as multimorbidity. Chronic disease therefore may also have the presence of co-related disability manifestation as part of the lived experience of chronic illness.

Reflection

1. How do beliefs affect communication with people with chronic illness?
2. How do your first-hand experiences, values and beliefs impact the care you give?

Indigenous populations

Worldwide, there are vast disparities in the health of Indigenous people and their subsequent experiences of chronic disease and/or disability, as compared with that of non-Indigenous people (WHO, 2008). This disparity is attributable to a life expectancy that is 10–20 years less than for the main population. A substantial proportion of Indigenous people suffer from malnutrition and communicable diseases. Indigenous peoples' ill-health is further exacerbated by damage to their habitat and resource base (WHO, 2008).

The health disparity presented worldwide continues to also be true for both Australian and New Zealand Indigenous populations. They are more likely to have an increased presence of chronic disease; to be less healthy; to die at a much younger age; and to have a lower quality of life than non-Indigenous people (AIHW, 2020; Ministry of Health, 2012).

Reflection

1. What are the health disparities in Australia and New Zealand for Indigenous people?
2. What factors contribute to Indigenous people having limited access to health services?
3. Why do Indigenous people distrust healthcare?

Inquiry

Chronic conditions are often associated with some level of disability but not always. It is said '**people with chronic disease often believe they are free from the disease when they have no symptoms**'.

1. Is this statement true?
2. Can an individual with chronic illness live a normal life?
3. What is the relationship between chronic illness and disability?
4. What is an example of a chronic illness with disability?

Action

1. Consider how you would ensure within your clinical practice that you do not use preconceived perceptions of people with chronic illness and disability when you give care.
2. What are some helpful strategies for coping with the person having a chronic disease and disability?

3. How can you help someone to reflect on their lifestyle and the impact it has on contributing to their chronic condition?

Understanding chronic diseases and prevention

Most chronic diseases are the result of people's risk behaviours. Major risk factors include poor nutrition, physical inactivity, tobacco use and excessive alcohol consumption. Poor nutrition includes diet that is low in fruits and vegetables and high in sodium and saturated fats. Sugary drinks are the leading source of added sugars and that includes the adding of sugar, cream and ice cream to coffee and tea. Good nutrition on the other hand is essential to keeping current and future generations healthy across the lifespan.

Tobacco use is the leading cause of preventable disease, disability and death globally. It is important for people to eliminate exposure to second-hand smoke. How much physical activity depends on whether you are maintaining your weight or are trying to lose weight. Achieving and maintaining an appropriate weight includes healthy eating, physical activity, optimal sleep and stress reduction. The Blue Zones website reveals the countries where people live longest (bluezones.com).

Reflection

1. How do you see your role as an educator in caring for people with chronic illness and disability?
2. How do you see yourself as a health promoter?
3. How do you see your role as an advocate to support people to self-manage their disease and disability?
4. How do you see yourself as a champion in running programs for the community?

CHAPTER 2

Living with a person with disability

Nathan J. Wilson

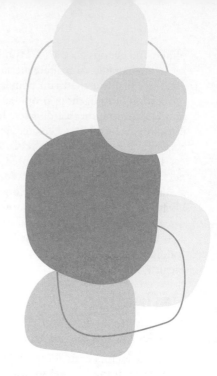

INTRODUCTION

This chapter will present short stories about three men who are living with a disability and disability-associated chronic illnesses. By engaging with these stories and the reflective activities in this chapter, the reader will become more acquainted with some of the issues facing people with a disability and will be better equipped to be a more responsive and adaptable health practitioner. Key issues are centred around activity and participation limitations due to disability, the intersection of chronic illness and disability, and a strong desire to achieve personal goals despite the daily challenges these men face. But first, a short introduction to the three men who have shared their stories.

Before you begin
Key contextual issues

- **The International Classification of Functioning, Disability and Health (ICF):** Central to the lives of all people with disabilities, including that of Aaron, Jamie and Grant, are the activity limitations, participation restrictions and intersecting health problems that result from having a physical disability. The ICF is a (2001) World Health Organization-endorsed framework for measuring both health and disability, and all health and social care workers should know about the framework as it helps to contextualise the often all-encompassing impact of having a disability. That is, a person's disability does not exist solely as an impairment to body function or structures – such as having a spinal cord injury resulting in quadriplegia – rather it is a dynamic interaction between health, personal and environmental factors, as illustrated in Figure 2.1 below. Importantly, the environmental factors are the barriers or facilitators that enable a person to live independently in society.

- Before reading on, think about someone you know with a disability and use the ICF model illustrated in Figure 2.1 to get a detailed insight into the dynamic factors that are at play that disable the person. In particular, think about

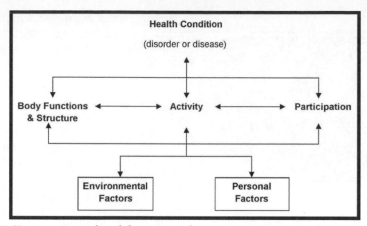

Figure 2.1 The ICF. (Source: *Reproduced from Towards a Common Language for Functioning, Disability and Health: ICF, The International Classification of Functioning, Disability and Health, Page No.9, 2002, WHO.*)

the environmental barriers and facilitators specific to this person. For example, if the person you are thinking about uses a wheelchair, what modifications can you identify – such as wheelchair ramps or accessible public transport – that promote their participation in society? Once you have listed these facilitators or barriers, think about what restrictions this would place on their activity or participation if they did not exist.

- **Terminology:** There are many terminology nuances within the disability field that are worth knowing as they are directly relevant to the holistic care and support that a person with a disability receives from health and social care workers. One main difference is between a lifelong and an acquired disability. For instance, Grant has an acquired disability as, prior to his spinal cord injury, he did not live with a disability at all and so most of his life experience was as a non-disabled person. Aaron and Jamie, on the other hand, have a global developmental disability as their disability occurred at birth and so has directly affected all of their developmental milestones. So, all three men have a physical disability, however Jamie and Aaron have always had a disability and, in addition, have a mild intellectual disability that is associated with their cerebral palsy. Note, however, that not all people with cerebral palsy have an intellectual disability, although they often co-occur (Wilson & Charnock, 2022).

- **Knowledge and attitudes of health workers:** The third, and final, vital contextual issue that you should consider relates to the knowledge and attitudes of others towards people with disabilities. Of note is that some of the main healthcare barriers and health disparities faced by people with disabilities are the knowledge gaps and sometimes negative attitudes of health and social care workers towards them. With respect to knowledge gaps and nurses, a recent literature review about registered nurses' perceptions of caring for someone with intellectual and developmental disability showed that they felt underprepared, faced communication barriers and were unsure about the role of family and/or paid carers (Lewis et al., 2017). This is important as feeling confident and competent to provide nursing care to an individual, regardless of any individual requirements, is vital for everyone. Notably, a very recent Australian survey of registered nurses showed that most had never received any education specific to people with intellectual and developmental disabilities and very few had been on a clinical placement during their education (Cashin et al., 2021). These knowledge gaps contribute to poor healthcare experiences by people with disabilities and are also associated with poor attitudes. For example, an integrative review by Desroches (2020) reported mainly negative attitudes by mainstream nurses, with limited knowledge and experience key factors.

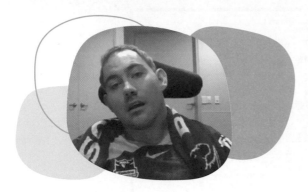

Aaron's story

 View Aaron's story or read his transcript.

Aaron is a man in his mid-thirties who lives in a supported accommodation facility with four other people with a disability. Aaron is a keen sports fan, in particular rugby league, and attends a day program two days a week where he participates in a range of life skills and social activities. Diagnosed with cerebral palsy at birth, Aaron also has a shunt for hydrocephalus which requires regular monitoring to assess for signs of a potentially fatal blockage. Aaron has a long-term goal to be an elite sports coach and has started on this journey by completing an online coaching course.

Aaron's story is filled with positivity that is grounded in the reality that life for Aaron is a 'big challenge'. Of note was Aaron's acute awareness of his shunt and the need for regular reviews to avoid the shunt blocking, as it did so often when he was a baby. Hydrocephalus is when the cerebrospinal fluid accumulates within the brain, putting pressure on the skull, and was first noted by Hippocrates in the 5th century BC (Aschoff et al., 1999). The shunt helps to drain the fluid away from the brain, usually into the abdominal cavity, to reduce the intracranial pressure. Aaron also talked about being teased when he was at school, but he managed to cope with this by blocking it out. Having set himself the goal of being an 'NRL Coach', and noting that it was an ambitious goal, Aaron had undertaken an online coaching course. What stands out is that despite a clear interest and the realisation of the many barriers he faced, Aaron did not have a job of any sort and attended a disability-specific day program two days a week where the focus was not about transitioning to work, that the services offered to Aaron were

limiting when compared with his ambitions. Also, that Aaron, a seemingly articulate man with a lot to offer, did not talk about having had a paid job before in his life.

Reflection

1. Would you say that Aaron has reached his potential in life? If not, what might be missing for him and how might he be supported to realise this, and by whom?

2. What impact do you think Aaron's healthcare experiences as a child influence his approach towards his healthcare needs today?

3. Aaron stated that he coped with being teased when he was younger, however this was at a time when inclusive education was in its infancy. Do you think that school children with disabilities in today's inclusive settings experience teasing and bullying? If so, how might that impact their overall health and wellbeing?

4. In your opinion, what might the role of a nurse who specialises in working with people with intellectual and developmental disability play in Aaron's life to help him achieve his goals?

Inquiry

1. The Professional Association of Nurses in Developmental Disability Australia (PANDDA) Inc. is the only Australian professional association for nurses that specialise in the area of intellectual and developmental disability. PANDDA recently revised its practice standards which offer a detailed insight into the biopsychosocial role of nurses, and how they work with individuals and their families in an individualised and person-centred way. Read these standards when you reflect on the above questions, as they will help you to conceptualise the broad scope of practice of these specialised nurses. They can be accessed at this website: www.pandda.net

2. There are mixed reports about the prevalence of bullying people with a disability, but the evidence is clear that bullying can have a significant impact on the person. Read this interesting article, 'Bullying adolescents with intellectual disability' (Christensen et al., 2012), which refers to people with a disability being bullied and bullying others. In particular,

take note of one of the opening background points that bullying has not been widely studied in people with intellectual disability.

Action

1. If you were working with Aaron, what might be the next steps that you could do in order to support Aaron to increase his activity and participation in sports coaching?

2. Once you have decided upon a step that you can take, what members of the multidisciplinary team would you engage with to support Aaron to participate more fully and independently in some form of sports coaching?

3. How do individual funding models work and how might they be used to support Aaron to get more involved in sports coaching?

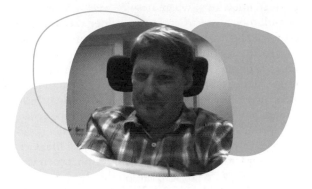

Jamie's story

 View Jamie's story or read his transcript.

Jamie is in his mid-fifties and lives in the same supported accommodation facility as Aaron. Jamie attends the gym once a week where he focuses on muscle strengthening and flexibility as a therapy for his cerebral palsy. Jamie also attends a day program two days a week which is focused on life skills. Jamie has a desire to find a partner and to have children. In addition, Jamie is interested in getting a 'proper' job as he wants to work. In addition to having some underlying mental health issues, Jamie also lives with gastro-intestinal problems that are associated with having cerebral palsy.

Jamie's story covers a number of topics, but his desire for a job and a partner stand out as unfulfilled life aspirations. In Australia there are two main types of employment for people with disabilities: 1) an Australian Disability Enterprise (ADE), previously referred to as sheltered employment, such as a factory; and 2) open employment, whether supported or independent, in the mainstream employment market. Jamie also talked about his exercises at the gym, where he is supported to work on his muscles, in particular to improve their tone. Although Jamie mentioned that he wanted to walk, it is not possible from his story to know if this is possible or whether the gym exercises were to maintain his current level of function to avoid deterioration as he ages. Such exercise and mobility are crucially important for people who use a wheelchair, as sedentary activity has an impact on many body systems, most notably the gastrointestinal system, where movement through daily activity and mobility is one part of the bowel's way of functioning in a healthy manner. For many people with a disability, however, gyms have many environmental and social barriers, such as the many unwritten social rules at the gym that are particularly challenging for people with intellectual disability. A recently published Delphi study that sought to identify the essential elements of an accessible fitness centre indicated that environmental adaptations and individualised preparations for exercises were important, along with responses to emergencies (Hong et al., 2022).

Reflection

1. Now in his mid 50s, do you think that Jamie might have outgrown a disability day program that focuses on life skills and recreation?

2. What is your judgement about the employment prospects for Jamie, in terms of both type (ADE or open employment) and tasks?

3. What would be the most significant barriers for Jamie to get a job in either an ADE or the open employment market?

4. What are the main health and wellbeing benefits to being in some form of employment?

Inquiry

1. There are many published examples of how to make information or environments more accessible to people with disabilities. Excellent examples of how to make health information more accessible can be found in the Books Beyond Words series, where topics include going to the hospital and preparing for

testicular screening. Here is the link to the website where you can find more information: booksbeyondwords.co.uk

2. The Council for Intellectual Disability also provides some guidelines on how to make environments more accessible. Here is a link to its guidelines for making gyms more accessible: https://cid.org.au/our-stories/accessible-gyms-and-how-to-enjoy-them/

3. Have a read of the article 'An evaluation of employment outcomes achieved by transition to work service providers in Sydney, Australia' (Xu & Stancliffe, 2019), which explores outcomes from a transition-to-work program for young adults with disabilities leaving high school in the state of New South Wales. Note the differences between the outcomes based on the size of the service and the implied expertise of the service.

Action

1. If you were working with Jamie, what might be the next steps that you could do in order to support Jamie to identify some opportunities towards his goal of participating in employment?

2. Thinking over these opportunities, what members of the multidisciplinary team would you engage with to increase the chance of Jamie's goals being realised?

3. How do individual employment funding models work in your region, and how might they be used to support Jamie?

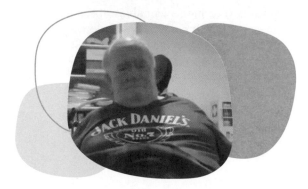

Grant's story

 View Grant's story or read his transcript.

Grant is a man who sustained a spinal cord injury some six year ago after a fall at his home in a regional area. Grant now lives in a major city in a supported accommodation facility. At one stage only being able to move one of his great toes after his injury, Grant is now able to walk a few steps with support. Although Grant has a very positive outlook on life, he does miss his old social networks and being able to tinker with his cars. Grant has ongoing problems with bladder infections where he accesses weekly care from a registered nurse to prevent hospitalisations for acute exacerbations of chronic bladder infections.

Grant's story is somewhat different to that of Aaron and Jamie's as his physical disability was quite recently acquired in adulthood. This means that most of Grant's life has been as a non-disabled person where the barriers to activity and participation are either absent or comparatively minor. The most important health issue facing Grant was recurrent bladder infections, where despite weekly visits by a community nurse to conduct bladder washouts, he estimated he was still hospitalised for acute infections two to three times per year. Hunter and colleagues (2013) conducted a literature review exploring long-term bladder drainage and noted that although there were many studies reporting clinical urology outcomes, few studies focused on the lived experiences of bladder drainage, such as daily management, satisfaction, stoma and skin care or quality of life. Certainly, for Grant, spending time in hospital each year would have a major impact on his health-related quality of life. A stand-out issue for Grant was his loss of independence and although not being able to swipe away a mosquito on your head would be extremely frustrating, perhaps the biggest impact was social isolation and the loss of friends. Although Grant did talk about befriending the neighbours, he also mentioned attending a disability-specific social group where he went on occasional outings.

Reflection

1. Is Grant's current social life, as described by him, as good as it might get or are there other ways that Grant might be supported to broaden his social networks?

2. What impact might a wider and more dynamic social life have on Grant's wellbeing, in particular his sense of loneliness, depression and isolation?

3. What are the main barriers that Grant faces if he wants to expand his social network and participate in activities outside the disability-specific services he currently accesses?

Inquiry

1. Men's Sheds are an Australian-inspired social space where mainly older retired men get together to socialise as they work on a range of practical projects such as woodwork or metalwork (Wilson & Cordier, 2013). A number of recent Australian studies have explored how men with disabilities have been supported to access Men's Sheds, thus widening their social networks and benefiting from greater activity and participation in terms of both their physical and their mental health. Read the following articles to gain a deeper understanding of how people with disabilities can be supported to participate in mainstream, rather than disability-specific, social groups: 'Men's Sheds: Enabling environments for Australian men living with long-term disabilities' (Hansji et al., 2015); 'A case study about the supported participation of older men with lifelong disabilities at Australian community-based Men's Sheds' (Wilson et al., 2015); 'Men with disabilities: A cross sectional survey of health promotion, social inclusion and participation at community Men's Sheds' (Wilson et al., 2016).

Action

1. If you were working with Grant, what might be the next steps that you could do in order to support Grant to identify some opportunities, such as Men's Sheds, in his community, to broaden his social network and engage in meaningful participation?

2. If you were to support Grant to attend a local Men's Shed, what members of the multidisciplinary team would you engage with, and why, to make this a success?

3. How do individual social inclusion funding models work in your region, and how might they be used to support Grant to attend a Men's Shed?

A FINAL WORD

This chapter has focused on the stories of three men, and taken the reader on a journey that is centred in the interaction between impairment, activity and participation, in order to illustrate how health and wellbeing outcomes are far more than just being physically healthy. All three men described having a good life, but noted areas of their life that could be improved with the right kind of support at the right time. The ICF framework has been introduced and all health and social care workers should be aware of this dynamic framework and how the experience of disability extends well beyond an individual's diagnosis or impairment.

CHAPTER 3

Living with rehabilitation

Michelle Stubbs

INTRODUCTION

This chapter contains two stories that describe the different experiences of people who have required rehabilitation services. The two cases offer individual perspectives on rehabilitation. The first relates to a person with a lifelong disability who needs rehabilitation to maintain as much functionality as possible to live her optimal life, and the second relates to an individual who has achieved a return to full functionality. While their individual goals may seem different, the need for rehabilitation is key for both people to achieve their desired outcomes.

Before you begin

According to the World Health Organization, globally there are an estimated 2.4 billion people currently living with a health condition that benefits from rehabilitation. The definition of rehabilitation is 'a set of interventions designed to optimise functioning and reduce disability in individuals with health conditions in interaction with their environment'. As a nurse you may think of rehabilitation as a health intervention used to help people 'recover' from a critical incident, whether this may be surgery, trauma or a medical cause such as a stroke or myocardial infarction. As you can see from the above definition, however, there is another function of rehabilitation, which is basically to help people with a chronic, incurable disease to maintain optimum function to enable them to live the best life they can with their disability.

- Have you ever thought about the use of rehabilitation in relation to long-term debilitating disease?

- What sort of complex medical needs might require an individual to need lifelong rehabilitation?

- How might the motivational needs of each end goal of rehabilitation differ? While it is comparatively easy to think about how to motivate a person to work towards full recovery over a relatively short time frame, have you considered how you might help support and motivate someone who is needing rehabilitation to try and stop any further limitation of their activities and lifestyle?

- How does an individual's motivation potentially affect the outcome of rehabilitation?

- How might a person's location impact on their ability to access rehabilitation services?

- How does family support impact on the ability of a person to access rehabilitation services?
- How does a person's financial situation impact on their access and utilisation of rehabilitation services?

Rehabilitation overview

Put simply, rehabilitation helps any individual to be as independent as possible in everyday activities and enables participation in education, work, recreation and meaningful life roles, such as taking care of family. It does so by addressing primary disease, illness or injury and improves the way an individual functions in everyday life, supporting them to overcome difficulties with thinking, seeing, hearing, communicating, eating or moving around. Rehabilitation might also help people to get moving again, regain their strength, relearn skills or find new ways of doing things. Anybody may need rehabilitation at some point in their lives, following an injury, surgery, disease or illness, or because their functioning has declined with age.

Rehabilitation services

Rehabilitation services are specialist healthcare services that help a person regain physical, mental and/or cognitive (thinking and learning) abilities that have been lost or impaired as a result of disease, injury or treatment. Rehabilitation services help people return to daily life and live in a normal or near-normal way. These services may include physiotherapy, occupational therapy, speech and language therapy, cognitive therapy and mental health rehabilitation services.

Rehabilitation services may be short-term, long-term or episodic depending upon the nature of the person's condition. While the demand for rehabilitation spans all ages, it increases with age. Older people are proportionally the largest group accessing these services. Central to the provision of rehabilitation services is the collaboration between multidisciplinary teams, patients and carers. This collaboration guides the development and implementation of care plans, and the process of reviewing a patient's progress against stated goals. Quality rehabilitation activities are patient-focused, educating and enabling patient self-management and taking into account the experiences of patients and those who care for them.

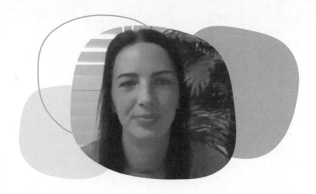

Bonnie's story

 View Bonnie's story or read her transcript.

Bonnie Lauder is the mother of a child with progressive scoliosis. Bonnie describes the difficulties of navigating the health system with a complex and rare rehabilitation issue. Bonnie's daughter needs lifelong rehabilitation to maintain optimal health while co-existing with a lifelong degenerative illness.

Reflection

What is your understanding of the emotional impact that is associated with caring for a child with a chronic and continuing illness such as progressive scoliosis? Does having scoliosis as a child pose an increased risk of health problems and reduced quality of life as an adult? You may wish to review your understanding of progressive scoliosis and the burden it places on carers of people diagnosed with the disease. You may also like to examine pathophysiology, symptoms and types of scoliosis.

1. As a parent how do you think you would feel if your child had a lifelong need for rehabilitation services?
2. Think about how this would impact on your ability to work, to care for any siblings, to have the time, money and energy to be able to do things for your own physical and mental health.
3. If you were caring for someone with scoliosis and the Schroth Method was part of their rehabilitation program, what would your role be?

You might like to research the biopsychosocial model of the disease and explore what government initiatives are currently available for carers of people with a chronic condition or disability.

1. List the challenges faced by Bonnie and her daughter.
2. What services are available to help Bonnie from a psychological and financial perspective?
3. How likely do you think it will be that either Bonnie or her daughter might become depressed?

You might like to research different rehabilitation services for particular conditions. For example, you could research the Stroke Recovery Association in relation to stroke rehabilitation, or the Victorian Mental Illness Awareness Council in relation to psychiatric rehabilitation.

1. Bonnie talks about a disconnect between public and private services. Are different services provided to people undergoing rehabilitation in these different sectors? Think about your understanding of each sector.

2. As a carer for a person undergoing rehabilitation, what would be your first action if rehabilitation services were not available in your area?

3. What is the role of the General Practitioner in organising rehabilitation services?

   Think about the role of rehabilitation specialists. As a carer, if you recognised that the treating rehabilitation specialist was underperforming in their duties, what would you do?

4. Do all people undergoing rehabilitation have access to a case manager?

5. What is the role of a case manager?

6. Does the role of the case manager differ between public and private sectors as well as rehabilitation programs?

7. Bonnie voices that future carers should advocate. What is your understanding of advocacy? Have you ever advocated for someone in the past? Would you be able to advocate better if you were a member of a support group?

8. What can support groups offer carers of a person undergoing rehabilitation?

9. Bonnie also talks about setting goals. How are rehabilitation goals set and by whom?

10. What support groups do you know of that help carers of long-term rehabilitation clients?

    Bonnie suggests getting copies of everything as 'sometimes connections aren't made' and 'documents aren't forwarded'. How do you think this lack of effective communication between variable health professionals would impact on a person with low health literacy?

11. How does the carer of a person undergoing rehabilitation communicate that established rehabilitation goals are unattainable or not specific enough?

12. In what ways can a carer of a person undergoing rehabilitation look after themselves? What is the definition of self-care?

Inquiry

1. SpineUniverse is a leader in spine education for people with scoliosis, providing clear and direct information on conditions including sciatica, spinal stenosis, ankylosing spondylitis, spondylolisthesis and scoliosis. The SpineUniverse website offers content developed and vetted by a distinct team of experts in their fields, including orthopaedic surgeons, neurosurgeons, pain management physicians, physical therapists and other spine specialist clinicians. At this point you may like to take the time to access the SpineUniverse website and become familiar with the information located under the conditions and treatments tab: https://www.spineuniverse.com

2. The Australian Government's Department of Social Services details its mission to improve the wellbeing of individuals and families in Australian communities. The Department of Social Services is overseen by several Ministers. Within this department, Ministers have areas of responsibility; for example, Minister for the National Disability Insurance Scheme. Overall, the Department of Social Services helps to support families and children through programs and services as well as benefits and payments. At this point, you may like to take the time to access the Department of Social Services website and become familiar with information located under the disability and carers tab: https://www.dss.gov.au

3. The Agency for Clinical Innovation (ACI) is the lead agency for innovation in clinical care. The ACI brings together patients, clinicians and managers to support the design and implementation of innovation in health care. The vision of the ACI is to create the future of health care, and healthier futures for the people of New South Wales. For carers, the ACI can be of assistance if transition from paediatric to adult healthcare services is required. The ACI website offers information concerning clinical networks, industry/education events and state-wide programs.

Take time now to visit the ACI website. Explore the information available under the clinical networks tab. Familiarise yourself with material relating to chronic and long-term care as well as rehabilitation (under the Trauma, Pain and Rehabilitation heading): https://aci.health.nsw.gov.au

4. The Scoliosis Support Network is a support group that shares support and encouragement between families of those affected by scoliosis. This group was created on Facebook in 2010 with the aim of providing a safe place for people to connect and support each other. The Scoliosis Support Network currently has about 8000 people from around the world either liking or following the page. There are several benefits of a support group on social media including increased emotional support, information support and social companionship. Furthermore, people are more likely to have improved quality of life, be engaged in their care and have lower rates of depression – all by interacting with people who suffer from the same condition. With social media's growing influence on people, it's no surprise that it has a place in health care. More and more patients/people are connecting with others going through the same health issues – and learning how to better advocate for themselves from each other. You may wish to visit this support group on Facebook and scroll back through past posts: https://www.facebook.com/Scolipals

Action

1. Describe the different reasons people may be needing rehabilitation services. Think about how the different potential outcomes of rehabilitation will impact on the patients and carers. Don't forget to consider the implications of the potential impact on these individuals if the care is not timely and available.

2. What ancillary support services might you be able to enlist for those individuals who are struggling to access rehabilitation services, whether this is financial, locational or related to family issues?

3. What do you know and understand about human motivation? Consider if this is an area of knowledge you feel would be beneficial to learn more about. How do you think understanding human motivation might help you to help your patients?

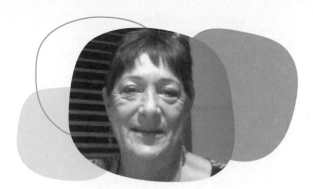

Jacqueline's story

 View Jacqueline's Story or read her transcript.

Jacqueline Brewer is a 65-year-old woman, who has undergone bilateral knee replacements and with the help of rehabilitation services has regained full mobility.

Reflection

Jacqueline is a person who is highly motivated to recover from her surgery. She is accustomed to being a very physically and capable individual and has every reason to believe that following rehabilitation her life will return to pre-disease function. What have you learned from listening to Jacqueline?

1. Reflect on how this very favourable outcome is likely to impact on her desire to engage fully with rehabilitation requirements.

2. What do you understand about how intrinsic and extrinsic motivation may assist a person's recovery?

3. Do you think Jacqueline is highly motivated? Why do you think she might be highly motivated? Think about whether or not Jacqueline is accustomed to being highly mobile and self-sufficient.

4. In a hospital setting, do you think the patient's preoperative baseline health status might be a factor in whether they are highly motivated to attend their rehabilitation requirements?

5. List other reasons why a person may not be so highly motivated. Consider pain tolerance.

6. During her interview, Jacqueline mentions pain and pain management. Reflect on your understanding of pain and treatment of pain.

Do you think Jacqueline has suffered from chronic pain prior to surgery?

7. Are there differences in how chronic and acute pain is treated?

8. Can Jacqueline expect to be pain free when rehabilitation is completed? At this point in time, you may like to research current pain management guidelines for chronic and acute/postoperative pain.

9. Think about how pain is assessed both inside and outside a hospital setting?

10. What is your understanding of multimodal pain relief?

11. Think about poorly controlled postoperative pain. Why is adequate pain relief important during the immediate postoperative period?

12. How does the postoperative treatment impact on mobility status and the development of chronic pain?

13. Rehabilitation may be classified as either prehabilitation (prior) or rehabilitation (thereafter). The topic of prehabilitation and rehabilitation is of interest to healthcare systems to enable evidence-based decision making regarding which interventions should be offered to people undergoing total knee arthroplasty (replacement) to achieve best clinical outcomes, reduce avoidable complications or joint failures, and be cost- and resource-effective for the healthcare services, patients and their caregivers. Can you identify what factors indicate that inpatient rehabilitation would achieve better outcomes for an older person with limited social support and existing comorbidities?

14. Which factors impact patient-related outcomes following hip or knee arthroplasty?

15. What factors influence the choice of setting for rehabilitation after knee and hip arthroplasty?

16. How effective is inpatient rehabilitation following hip or knee arthroplasty compared with outpatient rehabilitation, community rehabilitation, home-based rehabilitation and no rehabilitation?

17. Explore the total journey from initial consultation with a surgeon to long-term joint-replacement health. Before you explore the total journey, think about the burden of time that healthcare appointments place on people. Also think about living each day with diminished levels of functioning.

18. Think about the preoperative phase. Should a person undergoing a total knee arthroplasty worry about their weight, blood pressure, diabetes and smoking? If yes, who is the best healthcare clinician to help with these issues?

19. Consider surgery. What types of anaesthetic options are available for people undergoing total knee arthroplasty? What are the risks of surgery?

20. Reflect on the postoperative phase. If postoperative recovery is not going as well as expected, what actions should be undertaken? Would unplanned complications impact the mental health of a person undergoing rehabilitation?

21. Jacqueline mentions that 'if you undertake rehabilitation, you will recover really well'. Take a moment and think about what recovery means. In relation to a total knee replacement, when are you considered to be recovered? In terms of rehabilitation, when does rehabilitation stop? Is rehabilitation a life-long course of care?

22. Consider the actions to be taken when either rehabilitation goals have been reached or progress is not being made during rehabilitation. Should a person undergoing rehabilitation talk to their surgeon, general practitioner or physiotherapist about this? Is this a problem for one particular healthcare professional or is this a team problem?

23. Consider multidisciplinary teams in rehabilitation. What healthcare professionals are vital to an orthopaedic rehabilitation team?

24. Are the same healthcare professionals necessary in rehabilitation teams for other conditions?

25. Reflect on other conditions or diseases. What are the components of rehabilitation interventions for stroke, brain injury and spinal cord injuries?

Inquiry

1. The Australian Commission on Safety and Quality in Health Care is a corporate Commonwealth entity under the Public Governance, Performance and Accountability Act 2013. The Commission was established as a result of the federal government passing the National Health Reform Act 2011. The Australian Commission on Safety and Quality in Health Care is jointly funded by all governments on a cost sharing basis, and the

Commission's annual program of work is developed in consultation with the Australian, state and territory Health Ministers. One role of the Commission is to develop Clinical Care Standards. You may now wish to reflect on your knowledge of policies and protocols surrounding osteoarthritis and total knee replacements. You can access further information about osteoarthritis of the knee and Clinical Care Standards at: https://www.safetyandquality.gov.au/sites/default/files/2019-06/oak_dst_final_june_3.pdf and Gold Coast Health: https://www.goldcoast.health.qld.gov.au/sites/default/files/TKR%20Patient%20Guide.pdf

2. *The Australian Journal of General Practice* aims to provide relevant, evidence-based, clearly articulated information to Australian general practitioners to assist them in providing the highest-quality patient care, applicable to the varied geographic and social contexts in which general practitioners work, and to all general practitioner roles as clinician, researcher, educator, practice team member and opinion leader. All articles in the journal are subject to peer review before they are accepted for publication. The journal is indexed in MEDLINE, Index Medicus and Science Citation Index Expanded. As the journal is open access, readership of the publicly available online version extends more broadly into the international healthcare and education sectors as well as patients and carers. You may wish to visit the journal website and read the below publications:

   - 'Symptom management for patients awaiting joint replacement surgery' (Wall et al., 2020): https://www1.racgp.org.au/ajgp/2020/july/symptom-management-for-patients-awaiting-joint-rep

   - 'Changes to rehabilitation after total knee replacement' (Sattler et al., 2020): https://www1.racgp.org.au/ajgp/2020/september/changes-to-rehabilitation-after-total-knee-replace

   - 'Pre-operative optimisation for hip and knee arthroplasty: Minimise risk and maximise recovery' (Wall & de Steiger, 2020): https://www1.racgp.org.au/ajgp/2020/november/pre-operative-optimisation-for-hip-and-knee-arthro

3. The Royal Australasian College of Surgeons, formed in 1927, is a non-profit organisation training surgeons and maintaining surgical standards in Australia and New Zealand. The Royal Australasian College of Surgeons is an umbrella organisation representing the interests of all Fellows in whatever specialty they practise. They provide continuous professional development, training and accreditation for surgeons. There are nine surgical specialties in Australia and New Zealand being: Cardiothoracic Surgery, General Surgery, Neurosurgery, Orthopaedic Surgery, Otolaryngology Head and Neck Surgery, Paediatric Surgery, Plastic and Reconstructive Surgery, Urology and Vascular Surgery. You may wish to visit the website and use the search bar to review freely available documents relating to total knee arthroplasty: https://www.surgeons.org/-/media/Project/RACS/surgeons-org/files/reports-guidelines-publications/surgical-variance-reports/2018-01-29_mbp_arthroplasty_final.pdf?rev=cad69a225fee486ead d75779bf7b8425&hash=8CC9E285C9E88644 0BCBA25A1A86F0ED

4. Another resource providing information comes from the Northern Sydney Local Health District. In collaboration with the New South Wales Government, they have produced an educational booklet titled *Advanced Recovery for joint replacements in Northern Sydney: Your guide to preparation and recovery (ADVANSYD Pathway)*. This booklet provides information about joint replacement surgery, and what people need to do before, during and after surgery. It is a great resource that healthcare professionals could advise patients to refer to throughout their journey. You may wish to visit the Healthtalk Australia website and familiarise yourself with the information they provide: https://www.nslhd.health.nsw.gov.au/MySurgeryJourney/Documents/NS11869B-E.pdf

5. Royal Rehab is Australia's leading provider of rehabilitation and disability services. Royal Rehab is located in the suburb of Ryde in Sydney, New South Wales, and was established over 120 years ago by an extraordinary woman named Susan Schardt. Royal Rehab is highly regarded for its specialist expertise in brain and spinal cord injury rehabilitation. It is also well known for its services surrounding supported accommodation and community services. Royal Rehab employs a multitude of clinicians including allied healthcare professionals. One goal of the skilled multidisciplinary team of healthcare professionals at Royal Rehab is to support people to achieve as

much independence and quality of life as possible. This includes assisting people to adjust to changed abilities, relearn skills and gain new ones, and reintegrate into their homes and the community. Please take a moment to review the content on their website and become familiar with the rich history of Royal Rehab and the work of Susan Schardt and review information on the website relating to orthopaedic rehabilitation medicine: https://royalrehab.com.au

Action

1. Explore the complete journey of undergoing a total knee arthroplasty as identified by Jacqueline throughout her video. After reading literature, do you have any question about total knee arthroplasty that remain unanswered?

2. Describe the importance and influence that motivation has on rehabilitation outcomes.

3. Do complications negatively impact a person's motivation and program completion rates of rehabilitation?

4. Think about your own learning and attitudes relating to the administration of pain relief. Do you work in an environment that is reluctant to give opioid medications for pain? Are you concerned the patient may become addicted? How do you differentiate between whether you give a patient opioids or non-opioid pain relief. Do you take a proactive or a reactive approach to post operative pain relief?

5. Consider the effectiveness of all settings of rehabilitation. Can you argue that an inpatient rehabilitation setting results in superior outcomes compared with those of home-based rehabilitation?

6. What is your role in the decision-making process surrounding appropriate rehabilitation settings for people undergoing total knee arthroplasty?

7. Reflect on your role as a nurse. What part do you play within a skilled multidisciplinary team of healthcare professionals in the rehabilitation setting? Do you think the role of the nurse is any less valuable than, say, a dietitian? How is respect shown within multidisciplinary teams? How might conflict with such a skilled and multidisciplinary team be overcome?

A FINAL WORD

As healthcare professionals, providing care to people recovering from injury or illness is understood to be an essential element in the rehabilitation journey. Patients may need rehabilitation for a multitude of reasons. For some it is the final stage of achieving complete recovery following a traumatic event or surgery. For others, though, it may be that they are striving to get as well as possible while knowing they are unlikely to ever recover fully, and for some it is a constant intervention to help them maintain the best health they can achieve. This means that as nurses we need to be aware of the reasons this person is in our care, and we need to tailor our care as always to the individual. Within a day's work, rehabilitation nurses may act as teachers, caregivers, collaborators and advocates. The importance of these roles should never be underestimated.

Working as a rehabilitation nurse is known to be one of the most rewarding careers in health care. You will frequently get to witness people push past their own limits and overcome exceptional odds. And as you typically work with the same people on a regular basis, you establish relationships with patients and their loved ones. Not only will you be seen as a caregiver and rehabilitation professional, but you'll also often be perceived as a friend and source of support during tough times. We hope you have enjoyed the experience of learning the ins and outs of rehabilitation in relation to orthopaedic rehabilitation and as the role of a carer of someone undergoing constant rehabilitation.

CHAPTER 4

Living with life-limiting illness

Sara Karacsony

INTRODUCTION

This chapter presents two distinct perspectives of living with or caring for a person living with life-limiting illness. As such, the chapter provides perspectives from a health service provider and a health service user who has embraced a role other than just that of a 'patient'. As you will see, understanding the needs, goals and wishes of patients is essential to their experience of illness and quality of care. The support needs of people living with life-limiting illness encompass a range of different services and resources and, since the COVID-19 pandemic, has seen telehealth become a viable and important way to improve access to healthcare services for patients living with life-limiting illness in regional and rural areas. New models of care have seen an increase in nurse-led care and the role of advanced practice nurses across the spectrum of patients' care needs as highlighted in both stories. This chapter focuses on adults with life-limiting or serious illness and these terms are used interchangeably in the chapter.

Before you begin

It is worthwhile examining your understanding of what constitutes life-limiting illness, including communicable and non-communicable diseases (NCDs), types of treatment options and medications that are available for people with serious illnesses, as well as the challenges of availability, access and affordability of treatments worldwide. You might also consider what the term 'seamless care' means and how the disruption to routine screening, diagnostic follow-up and treatments resulting from the COVID-19 pandemic is reported to have affected millions of people living with NCDs, such as cancer, heart diseases, chronic respiratory diseases, diabetes and other NCDs in accessing routine care and medicines. You might consider the specialty of palliative care and how and at what point the specialties of oncology, respiratory and renal medicine intersect with palliative care.

As a novice healthcare professional, think about how being diagnosed with a serious illness would change how you might think about your life. Do you think that a diagnosis of serious illness affects people in different ways? When you listen to the two stories, consider the importance of diagnostic testing and information provision as well as the early establishment and ongoing negotiation around goals of care. Reflect on your knowledge and skills to renegotiate these goals when a patient's treatment outcomes change and there is a need to refocus away from 'cure' or 'surveillance' to 'quality of life' and managing troublesome symptoms. Importantly, consider some of the skills that are needed to support effective communication. When should clinician–patient communication in serious illness take place?

The rise in NCDs (and some communicable diseases) as a result of ageing populations and resultant serious illnesses demands effective healthcare services that are accessible and affordable for millions of people worldwide. For example, the World Health Organization (WHO) reports that nearly every family globally is affected by cancer, either directly – 1 in 5 people are diagnosed with cancer during their lifetime – or as caregivers or family members (WHO, 2022b). Health-related suffering due to serious, life-limiting illnesses requires many different professionals with specialist skills, including medical, nursing, support workers, paramedics, pharmacists, social workers, dietitians, physiotherapists and volunteers. These skilled roles are required to address the multidimensional aspects of care that people need to alleviate suffering. Palliative care developed as a medical specialty for people diagnosed with cancer for whom no treatment options remained in the advanced stages of illness. The specialty of palliative care now focuses on the relief of health-related suffering across a wide range of illnesses, including cancer, chronic heart, kidney and liver disease, multiple sclerosis, Parkinson's disease, rheumatoid arthritis, neurological disease, dementia, congenital anomalies and drug-resistant tuberculosis (WHO, 2022a).

Across the world many millions of people do not have access to adequate treatment options or to palliative care and suffer distressing physical symptoms. Planning and controlling increasing symptoms early in the illness improves quality of life and relieves suffering and is seen as an ethical duty in the preservation of a person's sense of dignity (WHO, 2022b).

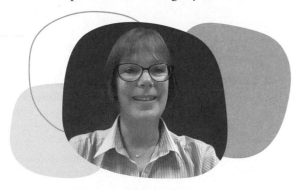

Rebecca's story

View Rebecca's story or read her transcript.

Rebecca Palmer is an endorsed Nurse Practitioner (NP) with the Supportive and Palliative Care Service in Nepean Blue Mountains Local Health District. Rebecca has been a registered nurse (RN) for over 30 years, working in the specialty of palliative care for over 20 years. Rebecca's role comprises predominantly clinical work within the community, including in-reach support for residential aged care services and the disability sector.

Reflection

After accessing the beginning of Rebecca's story, consider the following:

1. How does the scope of Rebecca's practice across the four domains of clinical, education, research and leadership enable her to work at the advanced practice level?

2. What do you perceive the value that the Nurse Practitioner (NP) role adds to healthcare services?

3. What communication issues might you find challenging if you were caring for a person diagnosed with serious illness?

4. What knowledge and skills do you think are important to be able to engage in Goals of Care conversations?

5. What do you understand the term 'supportive' to mean when Rebecca talks about her service?

6. Think about the potential challenges for a person trying to navigate the healthcare system. How might Rebecca enable this navigation?

7. What do you think are the benefits of normalising dying and death within communities and societies?

8. Rebecca describes the growth in consultations provided by the service. Consider why this has happened.

9. Rebecca emphasises the importance of self-care in her role. What steps do you, or might you, take to engage in self-care?

Inquiry

1. What are the key components of a Goals of Care conversation? How do you imagine you might do this? What is an Advance Care Plan? How is this different to a 'Goals of Care' conversation?

2. To help you, view Goals of Care resources on the following Australian websites:
   • Australian Commission on Safety and Quality in Health Care:

- https://www.safetyandquality.gov.au/our-work/comprehensive-care/essential-elements-comprehensive-care/essential-element-2-identifying-goals-care
- Caresearch Palliative Care Knowledge Network: https://www.caresearch.com.au/tabid/7455/Default.aspx
- palliAGED Palliative Care Aged Care Evidence: https://www.palliaged.com.au/tabid/4297/Default.aspx
- Advance Care Planning Australia: https://www.advancecareplanning.org.au/

Action

1. Review the Agency for Clinical Innovation (ACI) website on 'Virtual care: to safely connect health professionals with patients to deliver care when and where it is needed': https://aci.health.nsw.gov.au/statewide-programs/virtual-care

2. Consider if you would like to advance your career as a Nurse Practitioner. Review the Australian College of Nurse Practitioners website and learn more about Nurse Practitioners: https://www.acnp.org.au/aboutnursepractitioners

3. Palliative care in aged care is core business. Identify how the introduction of Palliative Care Needs Rounds are helping with the provision of palliative care in residential aged care facilities.

4. You might also like to check the Palliative Care Australia website for more information, including the Royal Commission into Aged Care Quality and Safety and valuable resources to support optimum palliative care in this setting: https://palliativecare.org.au/resource/palliative-care-in-aged-care/

5. Review other useful tools from Palliative Care Australia: https://palliativecare.org.au/, e.g.
   - 'Talking about Palliative Care': https://palliativecare.org.au/resource/talking-about-palliative-care/
   - What are common symptoms of people living in the advanced stages of their illness – when they are sick enough to die?

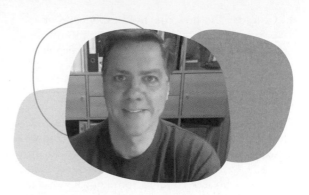

Peter's story

 View Peter's story or read his transcript.

Peter S lives in the Blue Mountains west of Sydney and is married with four sons. Peter has worked in various professional, student service roles in several of Sydney's major universities over the past 30 years. Just after Peter turned 60, he was diagnosed with stage 4 lung cancer.

Reflection

1. Without exception, no one is well prepared for the type of news that Peter received when he attended the Emergency Department (ED) at his local hospital with a vague sense of congestion in his chest. As he said, 'My experience is probably a very common one, in that you present for some medical attention, with no idea that [a diagnosis] of lung cancer is behind this thing.' Consider the profound shock that Peter describes on learning that his troubling respiratory symptoms might be due to 'congestive heart failure' or to 'cancer'. Reflect on what you know about these serious illnesses and your underlying assumptions about them, particularly their potentially life-limiting nature. How would you feel about such a diagnosis if it were you or someone close to you?

2. Reflect on Peter's description of being a 'super survivor' referring to the extraordinary success of the suite of targeted therapies for this particular cancer, and how this makes him feel. What support do you think is needed for 'survivors' of cancer?

3. Consider also how the 'lived experience' of people affected by cancer can help inform the needs and types of services for those people affected by cancer.

Inquiry

'One of the most common questions patients ask when they first learn that they have cancer is "but what caused it, doctor?" The most honest answer in many cases is "I don't know." This response can be reassuring for people who seek comfort from knowing that they are not themselves to blame, but may be disturbing for those who like explanation, and who find the concept of "fate" or a random event frightening. In circumstances where the answer is well known, as is the case of the cigarette smoker with lung cancer, a very sensitive reply is required' (Gaze & Wilson, 2003, p. 3).

1. At the turn of the 21st century, the authors of the above quotation wrote their book on Community Cancer Care. Since then, management and treatment of cancer has transformed. What was once a staple of surgery, radiation therapy, chemotherapy and other medical treatments, hormonal agents, biological response modifiers such as immunotherapy and targeted therapies have proliferated as a result of evidence-based clinical trials. Peter tells us that the treatment (Alectinib) he has received was developed in 2015 from Japanese research and made available on the (Australian) Pharmaceutical Benefits Scheme (PBS) in 2018. He also tells us that without access to the PBS, he would not have been able to afford this treatment, sold to him at less than half of 1% of its actual cost. What might this information tell us about the affordability of such treatments for the majority of the world's people?

2. In Australia, we benefit from many services that can assist people diagnosed and living with cancer to navigate cancer care and treatment options and support their decision making. Upon diagnosis, cancer care professionals typically offer people with cancer and their family/carers education and provide supportive materials, in hard copy and/or via website recommendations. Services may be provided by governments or not-for-profit organisations. Consider these sites, which provide information ranging from current clinical trials, personal and household changes, where to find nearby clinical support, and current treatment options:

   - eviQ: https://www.eviq.org.au/patients-and-carers
   - Australian Cancer Trials: https://www.australiancancertrials.gov.au/
   - Cancer Australia Treatment: https://www.canceraustralia.gov.au/impacted-by-cancer/treatment
   - Canrefer: https://www.canrefer.org.au/
   - Cancer Council: https://www.cancer.org.au/support-and-services

3. As you will learn from Peter's story, the continuous evolution of evidence-based treatments means some forms of cancer can be managed in this present day as a long-term chronic illness. Instead of focusing on dying and death, Peter tells a story that conceptualises his patient status not just as a 'survivor' – originally taken to describe a cohort of patients diagnosed with cancer who are followed over time to estimate the proportion surviving for a selected timeframe (e.g. 5 years) (Australia Institute of Health and Welfare, 2022) – but as a patient advocate, an active participant, decision maker – a patient partner – in the story of his illness. At this point you may want to read more about the involvement of patients in roles and with voices that are required to be heard across health systems.

4. As Peter's interview progresses, he talks about establishing priorities, finding the positives and getting involved in lung cancer research. What statistics does Peter share that provide perspective on his own story, considering men are far fewer than women in the patient partner arena even though lung cancer incidence is close to 50/50 between men and women?

5. How do you understand Peter's motivations and the benefits he derives from attending conferences and listening to the experts and bringing patients together?

6. At the beginning of this chapter, you were introduced to the role of the specialist palliative care nurse (Nurse Practitioner). You have also seen how varied and essential the nurse's role is in cancer care. In every cancer centre, specialist cancer nurses administer chemotherapy and other treatments, are trained in the management of vascular access devices, monitor and advise on treatment side effects, provide much information, support, counselling and referrals, and are often the first and last point of contact for patients and their families in treatment, managing symptoms and the trajectory of the illness. Like Peter, patients require many types of support. Notwithstanding the essential role of other members of the

multidisciplinary team in providing these various types of support: emotional, social, financial, spiritual – the psycho-social care provided by nurses is seen as just as essential to the person's wellbeing as good symptom control. Consider the importance of the psycho-social care nurses provide to patients.

Action

1. Peter describes a range of diagnostic tests and procedures that he undergoes to help with establishing a diagnosis and therapeutic interventions that help manage his symptoms. How important is our understanding of the levels of evidence required for a cancer diagnosis and cancer treatments?

2. **Diagnostic testing procedures**

   1. Identify some common diagnostic procedure that Peter refers to in this story and describe what these tests are.

   2. Consider the different timepoints when these tests are needed. How many times does an 'average' patient need to have these?

   3. Write this information in a table as demonstrated below:

Diagnostic testing	Example of when this test might be needed
X-ray	
CT scan	
PET	
MRI	
FISH	
IHC	

   4. What is the importance of diagnostic testing for Peter?

   5. What is a pleurodesis?

   6. What are the benefits of this intervention?

   7. How does Peter describe meeting the 'Thoracic Surgeon'?

3. As you go on to listen to Peter's story, he talks about the importance of building trust in the specialist doctors who recommend his treatment pathway, including his acceptance of being the first 'new' thoracic patient at the treating hospital. It is important to note how much trust Peter had to place in people he was meeting for the first time. We may take the 'expert' treating clinician for granted but what

is the basis of this trust? Why is trust so central to the healthcare and patient experience?

4. Consider now the steepness of the learning curve that Peter experienced from the point of considering his symptoms as indicators of 'lack of fitness' to the knowledge he gained about chest anatomy, diagnostic procedures and targeted therapy in the search for a diagnosis.

   • How might you rate Peter's health literacy at the start of the search for a diagnosis on a scale of 1–10?

   • How might a person's own health literacy impact their perceptions of life-limiting illness?

   • Is it possible to imagine how improved health literacy might be a cause for regret or would the opposite apply?

5. Take some time now to learn about the global statistics related to NCD, such as cancer, and what this means for healthcare services. Visit the World Health Organization health topics and review current prevention and management of this second leading cause of death worldwide: https://www.who.int/health-topics/cancer#tab=tab_1

6. If you or someone you know has been diagnosed with cancer, you may like to take the first WHO global survey to better understand the needs of all those people affected by cancer, whether as a patient who has completed cancer treatment, current family caregivers or bereaved family caregivers. The survey is part of a broader campaign, designed with and intended to amplify the voices of those affected by cancer – survivors, caregivers and the bereaved – as part of WHO's Framework for Meaningful Engagement of People Living with Noncommunicable diseases (PLWNCDs).

7. Investigate the decision-making processes that determine which medicines are listed on the PBS. What does this authority do? As Peter explained, the new treatments of cancer care have the potential to improve survival and quality of life of patients, but these treatments are expensive. How is cost effectiveness measured for new treatments, therapies and technologies?

8. Peter describes being a 'super survivor' – how does he consider his priorities? Take a look at some of the ways that patients can find the 'positives' in their illness? Review *Conquer* magazine and the stories of cancer patients who have become the experts in their own care.

A FINAL WORD

'A generation ago, most patients suffered in silence and ignorance, but today's patient is well informed and enquiring. This is due in part to those charitable bodies which provide a large amount of very high-quality information about cancer and its treatment and seek to empower the patient to be an equal partner in the therapeutic relationship; and partly to the way in which the "information super-highway" has made access to information from so many different sources available to so many' (Gaze & Wilson, 2003, p. 279).

While this is true in part, consider the role of the many, varied healthcare professionals in the stories shared by Peter and Rebecca who help to translate information, interpret diagnostic results and recommend treatments and who are able to hold meaningful conversations and build trusting and genuine relationships in a climate of complex, emotionally charged and deep uncertainty for patients and families. The experience of being a 'patient' requires an understanding that 'one patient's experience may say nothing about another's'.

We hope you have acquired some valuable learning and new insights as well as enjoyed listening to our storytellers.

CHAPTER 5

Living with depression

Robert Batterbee

INTRODUCTION

This chapter will explore caring for depression from the perspective of three clinicians working in very different areas of health care. All three clinicians will answer questions relating to their experiences of working within the context of contemporary Australian health and social care services. The aim is to explore the issues that impact the clinician, and their perception of the challenges faced by people who are living with depression.

Before you begin
How our beliefs and assumptions influence practice

It's important for clinicians to always be critically reflective in their practice. This involves being aware of all our preconceived assumptions, biases and beliefs about ourselves and others, and how these might influence our practice. Sometimes when our beliefs and assumptions are challenged by clinical situations, our emotions are triggered, and we react uncharacteristically. However, if we are aware of our biases, we can better understand the reactions that can influence our practice, and learn from these experiences. Before viewing the recording, or reading the transcripts from Karen Thomas and Clare Walters, please consider your views around the following questions, and the implications that these might have on your care.

- What is your opinion of people with a mental illness?
- Have you or any family member suffered with depression?
- Have your own experiences changed your perspective of mental illness?
- What are your beliefs about people who are homeless?

Low mood and depression: A brief clarification of concepts and terms

Depression is often a term that's used to describe the way we're feeling and doesn't always mean that we're suffering from a mental illness. 'I'm feeling a little bit depressed today' or 'I'm a bit low today' are statements often used to describe a mood state. A low mood is often thought to be normal if it's in the context of a challenging day ahead, a bereavement or receiving bad news. It's also very individual and linked to our personalities or social situations. Some people seem naturally happy and positive, while others are more negative and pessimistic.

When a low mood becomes depression, there are usually a few other features present. Physical symptoms commonly include disturbed sleep and appetite, reduced energy and loss of ability to focus. Thoughts become negative, and people start to ruminate and search for meaning to the situation, often concluding that they themselves are to blame. People start to avoid everything and lose interest in the things that used to make them feel happy. Finally, people with depression begin to isolate themselves. Their emotions become negative, and days become filled with sadness, frustration, fear and guilt. This is depression. Often the cause is known, sometimes it is not. Sometimes the depression will pass untreated, sometimes it will become acute and enduring.

When a low mood is present alongside physical illness or disability, it's important for the clinician to recognise when it's progressing towards depression. Depression can become more enduring than a primary illness. It can exacerbate an illness and negatively impact outcome, yet it can be easily treated.

Some added context

- **Emergency Department (ED):** The 24-hour emergency department (ED) in Australia and New Zealand is well known for treating acute, often life-threatening medical emergencies. ED is available to anybody that requires treatment and is also attended by people in crisis with mental health emergencies. These might be people who have attempted to commit suicide, who are simply in emotional crisis, who are acutely unwell with a mental illness, or who have been admitted to ED for another emergency physical treatment.

- **Mental Health Liaison Services:** Mental health liaison services are available in most emergency departments to provide assessment, initial care and access to specialist beds when required for people attending ED with mental and emotional emergencies. Clare refers to these as psychiatric liaison nurses (PLNs). PLNs are usually senior clinical nurses providing nursing care in ED. Some PLNs simply work as a 'liaison' nurse, or an interface between ED and Mental Health services, providing mental health triage and onward referral. Others are integrated into ED nursing teams and provide more comprehensive mental health nursing care across the department. There is usually one PLN working in each department who has access to an on-call psychiatrist and other team members if required.

- **'Revolving door' patients:** Clare mentions 'revolving door' patients. This is commonly used terminology referring to service users that frequently attend ED because their needs are unmet by other services. Clare speaks about unmet need in the community, but also in relation to mental health beds where people can be cared for appropriately as an inpatient.

- **Community nursing:** Community nurses provide an essential link in the healthcare management of people living with chronic illness in Australia and New Zealand. Community nurses work with patients and their families or carers providing nursing care to treat and prevent illness. Community nurses commonly treat people after discharge from hospital and work closely with general practice and other primary care services. Many community nurses specialise in a particular area of care; for example, wound management or palliative care. The community nurse requires a diverse set of clinical and interpersonal skills to treat a huge range of conditions in non-clinical and often challenging settings.

- **Rural and remote communities:** Community nursing in remote and rural areas of Australia presents a unique challenge to service delivery. Community nurses in remote areas often provide services that might be delivered by a multidisciplinary team in a metropolitan setting. Their skills are wide and diverse, treating conditions across the lifespan from birth to death. Community nurses often become a trusted and valued integral member of the community, just like the local GP, policeman and teacher.

- **Isolation:** As Holly mentions, it's sometimes a challenge for community nurses to access groups and other social resources for people living in rural areas. However, isolation can also be a behavioural symptom of depression as well as a geographical issue. Many people with depression stop enjoying doing the things that they used to do. To compound this further, the perception that depression is a sign of weakness often compels people to isolate themselves.

- **Nurse practitioner:** Nurse practitioners provide essential health care in a variety of clinical and community settings. In Karen's case, this is providing essential health care to the increasing homeless population in a metropolitan area of Perth, Western Australia. Nurse practitioners are often licensed to prescribe certain medications. They also liaise extensively with general practitioners, making recommendations for medications, treatment and onward referrals. Nurse practitioners therefore provide a link between primary care and the interface of the community where treatment is most needed.

- **Homelessness in Australia:** Over a quarter of a million people are assisted by specialist homelessness agencies in Australia each year: 39% of these people have been victims of family and domestic violence; over a third of all homeless people (39%) suffer with a mental illness, and 8.6% live with drug and/or alcohol issues (AIHW, 2022).

- **Homelessness and chronic illness:** People who are homeless have very complex healthcare needs that are often unmet by traditional services. Older people, who are more likely to suffer with chronic illness and disability, make up 9.3% or 25,300 of the homeless population seeking specialist support each year (AIHW, 2022). A report commissioned by the Australian Government and published by the Australian Housing and Urban Research Institute in 2014 suggests that many older homeless people suffer with chronic poor health, issues of substance misuse and institutionalisation (Petersen et al., 2014).

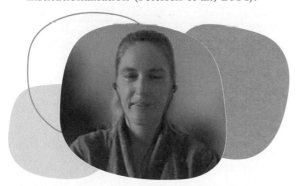

Clare's story

 View Clare's story or read her transcript.

Clare Walters is a clinical nurse working in a busy suburban emergency department in Western Australia.

Clare talks about her experience of providing emergency nursing care for people with depression as a primary and secondary issue. Clare shares her perspective as a clinician, reflecting upon the clinical and personal challenges that such a presentation can raise. She also shares her perception of challenges faced by her client group, and potential solutions to enhance care and improve service user outcomes.

Reflection

1. What in your opinion is the role of ED?
2. Is ED a provider of primary or secondary care?
3. Is ED an in-patient, or a community facility?
4. If there are gaps in primary-, community- or secondary-based care services, why are clinicians in ED more likely to be impacted?
5. In your opinion, what is the role of the comprehensive nurse in providing care for people with depression in ED?
6. After watching the video, you might also want to reflect again on your own assumptions about mental health. Also consider how it might feel to attend ED as a person in crisis living with depression.

Inquiry

1. The Nursing and Midwifery Board of Australia (NMBA) regulates the practice of nursing and midwifery in Australia by developing professional standards of practice for all comprehensively registered nurses. The NMBA states, in relation to all individuals being cared for, that:

   'These people may be healthy and with a range of abilities or have health issues related to physical or **mental illness** and/or health challenges. These challenges may be posed by physical, **psychiatric**, developmental and/or intellectual disabilities' (NMBA, 2016).

2. The full NMBA standards of practice can be accessed and reviewed here: https://www.nursingmidwiferyboard.gov.au/codes-guidelines-statements/professional-standards/registered-nurse-standards-for-practice.aspx

3. The following papers have also been selected for your consideration:
   - 'Principles for nursing practice: Depression' (Batterbee, 2022)
   - 'Repeat presentations to the emergency department for non-fatal suicidal behaviour:

Perceptions of patients' (Meehan et al., 2021)

- 'Perceptions of knowledge, attitude and skills about non-suicidal self-injury: A survey of emergency and mental health nurses' (Ngune et al., 2021)
- 'Emergency nurses' knowledge and self-rated practice skills when caring for older patients in the Emergency Department' (Rawson et al., 2017).

Action

1. Describe why it is important to understand the needs of people living with depression in any clinical setting.

2. Review your knowledge of the role of the comprehensive nurse in relation to people with mental health needs by reviewing the NMBA and ACMHN standards above.

3. Critically review the three above papers relating to mental healthcare in Australian emergency departments. Consider how this literature might inform your practice. Consider how ED can provide evidence-based care to people with depression.

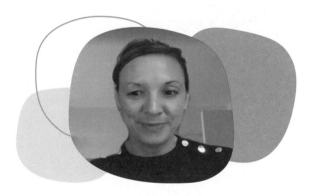

Holly's story

 View Holly's story or read her transcript.

Holly Clegg is a community nurse working in a regional area of Australia with limited community resources. Holly speaks about some of the practical and human challenges faced by the community nurse and their patients suffering with depression.

Reflection

1. What are the key skills needed for primary care and community nurses?

2. What role do community nurses provide in the provision of mental healthcare?

3. Why do you think that primary care nursing is such a rapidly growing workforce in Australia?

4. What would be the effects of an ageing population and associated chronic conditions on a person's mental health?

5. Consider this statement in the context of depression: 'general practice is the front door of all health services'.

6. You might also want to critically reflect upon your own beliefs and assumptions about the importance of emotional health care in community healthcare services. Do you or a relative have any experience of providing or receiving such care?

Inquiry

1. The Australian College of Mental Health Nurses (ACMHN) produces guidelines for mental health nursing care in Australia. This includes specialist psychiatric nursing care in mental health facilities, and mental health care provided by nurses in generalist environments, such as community nurses and those in general practice. In 2018 the ACMHN published Mental Health Practice Standards for nurses in Australian general practice in recognition of the growing role of the primary care nurse and changes to funding models (ACMHN, 2018). The full report and further best practice resources can be reviewed here on the ACMHN website: https://acmhn.org/best-practice-resources/#:~:text=The%20 Standards%20of%20Practice%20 provide,%2C%20and%20attitudes%20 (attributes).

2. The following papers have also been selected for your consideration.
   - 'An integrative review of primary health care nurses' mental health knowledge gaps and learning needs' (McInnes et al., 2022).
   - 'Help-seeking experiences of older adults with a diagnosis of moderate depression' (Polacsek et al., 2019).

- 'Impact of a mobile-based (mHealth) tool to support community health nurses in early identification of depression and suicide risk in Pacific Island Countries' (Chang et al., 2021).

Action

1. Describe why it is important to understand the needs of people living with depression in any clinical setting.

2. Review your knowledge of the role of the comprehensive nurse working in the community or primary care in relation to people with mental health needs by reviewing the ACMHN *Mental Health Practice Standards for nurses in Australian general practice* (ACMHN, 2018).

3. Critically review the three above papers relating to mental health in community and primary care services. Consider how this literature might inform your practice. Consider how primary care nurses can provide evidence-based care to people with mental health needs.

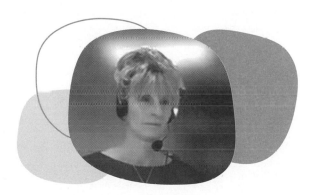

Karen's story

   View Karen's story or read her transcript.

Karen Thomas is a clinical nurse practitioner who works with the homeless population in Perth, Western Australia. Karen discusses some of the rewards and challenges faced by nurses working in this space, and shares her perception of some of the factors that present barriers to caring for her depressed service users.

Reflection

1. What are the key skills needed for a practitioner working with the homeless community?

2. What role do homeless workers provide in the provision of mental healthcare?

3. What do you think about the growing number of homeless people in Australia?

4. What do you think are some of the issues contributing to the problem?

5. What would be the effects of homelessness on a person's mental health?

6. You might also want to critically reflect upon your own beliefs and assumptions about homelessness by asking yourself the following questions
   - I believe that homelessness is …
   - I always assume that homeless people are …

Inquiry

The following papers have also been selected for your consideration.
- 'Homeless for the first time in later life: Uncovering more than one pathway' (Burns & Sussman, 2019)
- 'An effective homelessness services system for older Australians, AHURI Final Report No. 322' (Thredgold et al., 2019)
- 'Trajectories: The interplay between housing and mental health pathways' (Brackertz et al., 2020).

Action

1. Describe some of the emotional and mental challenges that might be faced by a person without a home.

2. Briefly research the services available for homeless people in your area.

3. Karen spoke about the difficulties of accessing mental health services for homeless people with depression. Critically review the following paper and consider how this might inform your practice: 'Service provision and barriers to care for homeless people with mental health problems across 14 European capital cities' (Canavan et al., 2012).

A FINAL WORD

Depression is often considered normal for people living in challenging conditions, or with a chronic health problem. However, depression can become a chronic and debilitating illness. Lots of people suffering with depression believe that to talk about their emotions is a sign of weakness and that they must not complain. Meanwhile, depression silently reduces their functioning – mentally, physically and socially. Yet in most cases, depression can be treated easily and successfully.

All healthcare professionals form an important link in the successful treatment of depression. Our clinicians' stories have illustrated that an understanding of depression and knowledge of the resources available for sufferers is fundamental to their role. The wellbeing of our patients and clients is our business, and timely intervention from all healthcare professionals can often provide a positive outcome.

CHAPTER 6

Living with dementia

Sara Karacsony, Sharon Andrews

INTRODUCTION

This chapter presents three distinct perspectives of living with or caring for a person living with dementia. The first story is presented by a person living with early onset Alzheimer's disease (Nell's story). The second story is provided by a caregiver to her mother diagnosed with dementia (Bronwen's story). The third story is provided by a lecturer in dementia care who is also a qualified occupational therapist (Melissa's story). The aim of the chapter is to explore key issues and considerations that can have an impact on people living with dementia, family caregivers and healthcare professionals.

Before you begin

It is worthwhile examining how our attitudes, beliefs and assumptions influence the way we think about dementia and shape care practice.

As a beginning healthcare professional, think about your own beliefs and assumptions about dementia. For example, do you think about dementia purely as a disease process? Do you think about dementia in terms of the impacts on the person living with a disease process? What have you observed in practice that reflects healthcare professional views or approaches to the care of people living with dementia?

A transformative theory of dementia care put forward by Tom Kitwood challenged the prevailing medical model that focused attention on the neuropathophysiology of the dementia illness and the disease-centric model (Kitwood, 1990). Instead, Kitwood proposed a new theory of dementia care that acknowledged the social and psychological

context of the person living with dementia. What followed was the development of the concept of personhood and person-centred care. According to Kitwood (1997, p. 8) personhood 'is a standing or status that is bestowed upon one human being by others in the context of relationship and social being. It implies recognition, respect and trust'. This new paradigm changed our thinking about dementia and taught us that people with dementia have psychological and social needs, that, if not met, can lead to distress. These needs, which are recognised as central to a person's wellbeing, include comfort, identity, attachment, occupation and inclusion (Kitwood, 1997). This then challenged thinking around care practices and caregiving for people with dementia from one of 'kindly oversight' (Kitwood & Bredin, 1992, p. 280) to one in which care focuses on promoting and maintaining wellbeing, even when a person is in the advanced stages of dementia.

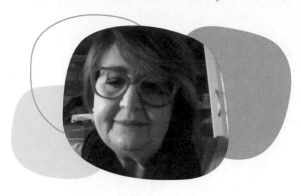

Nell's story

 View Nell's story or read her transcript.

Nell Hawe lives in northern New South Wales with her husband, son and poodle. Nell was diagnosed with early onset Alzheimer's disease in February 2020 after four years of 'fighting for a diagnosis'. Nell had begun to experience signs and symptoms of dementia but, unfortunately, her illness was not detected for some time. Nell is a passionate advocate for people living with dementia, especially in the context of timely diagnosis and dementia-care pathways.

Reflection

1. How do you think Nell's philosophy about living with her illness and '[dementia] coming along for the ride' reflects her personhood?

2. What are the challenges that Nell raises about living with dementia?

3. Can you think of any more to add to the list that Nell has not identified as challenges for herself? If so, add them now.

4. What does Nell mean when she talks about people being 'dementia friendly'?

5. What are your thoughts when you think about Nell's future? What might you think if a friend/relative told you they had been diagnosed with dementia?

6. Do you think Nell conforms to a stereotypical image of a person living with dementia?

7. Based on your thoughts on the previous question, how do you think this impacted Nell's experience of diagnosis?

8. Review what Nell's story about her knee replacement tells you about the knowledge, skills and attitudes needed by healthcare professionals?

9. What are the issues raised by Nell related to dementia training?

10. What do you think are the benefits of Nell engaging with the various dementia organisations (Forward with Dementia and Dementia Reframed)?

Inquiry

Considering Nell's experience from her initial presentation to her GP through to diagnosis, review the resources below that help explain younger-onset dementia and some of the symptoms that Nell speaks about.

- Information and support for people living with younger-onset dementia
- Memory changes
- Dementia and language
- Diagnosing dementia: early signs and symptoms

The Understanding Dementia MOOC will be another helpful resource for your inquiry.

Action

1. Review the Cognitive Decline Partnership Centre (CDPC) *Clinical Practice Guidelines* and *Principles of Care for People with Dementia*. Focus on the sections related to diagnosis, early identification and specialist assessment and identify how these may relate to your nursing practice.

2. Consider if you have observed similar instances in practice that corroborate Nell's story of her interaction with the pre-admission nurse in the surgical procedures ward.

3. Identify how that interaction could have occurred differently in the context of a person-centred approach.

4. Review the Global Dementia Charter: https://www.alzint.org/u/global-dementia-charter-i-can-live-well-with-dementia.pdf. This contains 10 points related to the perspective of a person living with dementia as they experience their journey.

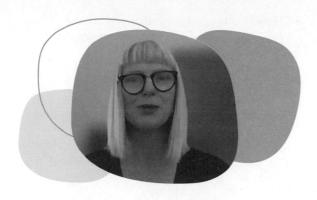

Bronwen's story

  View Bronwen's story or read her transcript.

Bronwen Fitzroy-Ezzy is a caregiver to her mother Heather. Bronwen has been providing care for several years. Heather is an 82-year-old lady who previously lived at home with the support of Bronwen, her husband and home-care services before moving to a local aged care facility. Heather was a high-school teacher, a very sociable lady and an avid reader. Bronwen and her husband live on the family farm and continue to be very active in Heather's care, frequently taking Heather out on excursions and for overnight stays at the farm.

Family caregivers are critical to care and quality of life of a person living with dementia. The role of family caregiver can be challenging with high rates of carer burden across physical, psychological and financial domains. It is important that factors that can ameliorate or exacerbate caregiver strain be identified. Optimal and successful caregiving requires building a network of support to provide care and engagement for the person living with dementia which, in turn, has positive effects on caregiving.

As an extension to Kitwood's person-centred care, Nolan and colleagues (2006) described 'relationship-centred care' with a more explicit focus on the centrality of relationships and the networks of interactions which support the person living with dementia and their caregiver. This framework comprises six senses that are considered to be essential to good relationships and quality care. These six senses are 'a sense of security – feeling safe'; 'a sense of belonging – feeling part of something, having a place', 'a sense of continuity – linking the past, the present and the future', 'a sense of purpose – having a goal to aim for', 'a sense of achievement – feeling you're getting

somewhere', and a 'sense of significance – to feel that you matter and are valued' (Nolan et al., 2004, 2006). Nolan and colleagues (2006) argue that good care can only be delivered when all of the senses are met, not just for the person with dementia, but also for the family caregiver and aged care staff. We will revisit the senses framework as we consider Bronwen's story. At this point you may want to read more about relationship-centred care in Nolan and colleagues' *The Senses Framework* (2006).

Reflection

As you listen to Bronwen or read her transcript you will recognise some of the senses from the work of Nolan and colleagues (2006) coming through her story.

1. Identify the parts of Bronwen's story that highlight the various senses (e.g. 'security', 'continuity', 'belonging').

2. What strategies does Bronwen use to promote the senses for Heather to maintain her personhood?

3. You may like to write this information in a table as demonstrated below

Senses	Example of strategy
Security	
Belonging	
Continuity	
Purpose	
Achievement	
Significance	

4. What are the benefits for Bronwen in continuing to ensure that Heather attends social events and maintains contact with her community?

5. How do you promote, or can you promote, the senses framework in your practice?

6. Bronwen talks about the importance of having support from other family members, who happen to be healthcare professionals involved with people living with dementia. It is interesting to note that Bronwen indicated that her journey would have been much more difficult without such support. What services and resources are you familiar with that can support the family caregiver of people with dementia?

7. There are a range of information resources and factsheets for family caregivers and friends that you may wish to review on the Dementia Australia website: https://www.dementia.org.au/resources/help-sheets#caring-for-someone-with-dementia.

8. Reflect on Bronwen's description of Heather becoming upset in the afternoons when in the aged care facility. Can you identify some possible antecedents to her distress, based on what you know about Heather?

Inquiry

As Bronwen's interview progresses, she talks about instances when Heather becomes distressed and upset. Behavioural and psychological symptoms of dementia (BPSD), also referred to as 'responsive behaviours' or 'changed behaviours', can impact on the person with dementia, family caregivers and care staff. One way of understanding changes to the behaviour of a person with dementia is to consider whether there is a 'trigger' or antecedent that is causing the change. These could be a need that has not been met [unmet needs such as hunger, loneliness, pain] and the behaviour is a form of communication. Or the change in behaviour could be due to the person with dementia having what is referred to as a lowered stress threshold, a result of the neurological impacts of the dementia. Identifying unmet needs (such as pain, hunger, social isolation) is critical to addressing the need and supporting the person with dementia.

Action

1. Take some time now to read and review some dementia guidelines. Dementia Support Australia has a range of resources that can assist you to understand BPSDs.

    • *Behaviour management: A guide to good practice*: https://www.dementia.com.au/resource-hub/behaviour-management-a-guide-to-good-practice

    • *A guide for family carers dealing with behaviours in people with dementia*: https://www.dementia.com.au/resource-hub/a-guide-for-family-carers-dealing-with-behaviours-in-people-with-dementia

    • Dementia Australia fact sheets on changed behaviour: https://www.dementia.org.au/resources/help-sheets#changed-behaviours-and-dementia

2. Identify some of the strategies that Bronwen and the staff at the aged care service used to support Heather when she became distressed. How do these strategies align with some of the best practice recommendations? Consider any other strategies that might be helpful.

3. How might you ensure that you adhere to best practice guidelines in your day-to-day care practice?

4. Bronwen describes being a caregiver as riding the roller-coaster and the importance of 'being in the moment … and enjoying the time you've got'. What are some strategies you can provide in your practice to support caregivers?

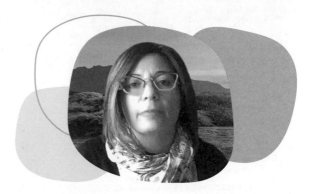

Melissa's story

 View Melissa's story or read her transcript.

Dr Melissa Abela began her work in dementia care as an occupational therapist and dementia consultant providing support and advice to people living with dementia at home and in residential aged care facilities in Sydney. Melissa's role focused on assessment of the person in their home environment and providing education and recommendations for home modifications to support the person to continue living at home. Melissa now lectures in dementia care.

Reflection

1. Melissa describes her assessment of factors in the home environment that may pose challenges for the person living with dementia. How might these factors pose challenges or barriers to a person's day-to-day experience?

2. What are some of the concerns that you might expect family caregivers to have for the person living with dementia at home?

3. What does Melissa do in her role that promotes safety and enablement of the person?

4. What do you understand by the term 'quality of life' in the context of Melissa's work?

5. Melissa emphasises throughout her story the importance of understanding the person, learning about who they are, their likes and dislikes, and discusses the dynamic nature of dementia that poses day-to-day challenges for care staff in residential aged care facilities. Melissa describes how staff might be missing a need that can lead to a 'changed' behaviour in the person. Consider the importance of knowing the likes and dislikes of a person living with dementia.

6. Why do you think a person's behaviours might change on a day-to-day basis?

7. Can you think of an example when you have seen someone whose behaviour has changed and you have not understood why? What new perspective might you have on this situation now?

Inquiry

1. Based on what you have now learned about best-practice dementia care, what do you think is encompassed by the 'excellent dementia care' that Melissa refers to? You might also like to consider how the built environment can be adapted to be supportive, familiar and therapeutic.

2. You can review the recommendations of the Royal Commission into Aged Care Quality and Safety (2021), specifically related to care of the person living with dementia in the residential aged care setting where dementia care is viewed as 'core business'. Importantly, the Commission draws attention to dementia care requiring a continuum of care from diagnosis through to palliative care, including prevention, primary care (such as provided by Melissa) and hospital care. View the Commission's recommendations: https://agedcare.royalcommission.gov.au/sites/default/files/2021-03/final-report-recommendations.pdf

3. Melissa describes her work in residential aged care facilities in supporting 'changed behaviours' in the context of the care environment. At this point, you might consider the impact that a transition from home to a care facility can have on the person living with dementia, as well as the impacts of caregivers. You have gained some understanding of this already from listening to Bronwen's story about Heather moving into a residential aged care facility. Read the following article that describes the experiences, unmet needs and health-related quality of life of family caregivers transitioning their care recipients with dementia into long-term care: 'Unmet needs and health-related quality of life of dementia family caregivers transitioning from home to long-term care: A scoping review' (Lee et al., 2022).

4. At the beginning of this chapter, you were introduced to the concept of person-centred care and, subsequently, to the concept of relationship-centred care. Consider the importance of information sharing as essential to the person's wellbeing.

5. Review the information provided in standard discharge documentation and consider whether this information is sufficient to provide a 'holistic' overview of a person living with dementia. Does it provide relevant personal and social information, which you have learned is vital to quality dementia care?

6. Take a look at some established initiatives to provide a more person-centred overview of the person for when the person is admitted to hospital and/or to a residential aged care facility:

   • https://www.cec.health.nsw.gov.au/improve-quality/teamwork-culture-pcc/person-centred-care/dementia-care

   • https://aci.health.nsw.gov.au/__data/assets/pdf_file/0008/285380/ACI-Agedcare-CHOPs-Sunflower.pdf

Melissa describes health professionals as requiring 'a thorough understanding of what the person may be experiencing as a result of changes in the brain'. Melissa goes on to discuss how essential education is for equipping healthcare professionals with the specialist knowledge and skills needed for quality care. These are equally important for job satisfaction and emotional health and wellbeing of healthcare providers.

Action

1. Take some time now to consider the knowledge, skills and attitudes that are required to provide optimum care for persons living with dementia. Write a summary of these key attributes.

2. Describe how you might build relationships and trust to explore emotions and difficulties of family caregivers presenting to aged care services.

3. Some of the physical effects of dementia include incontinence. This problem has the potential to

impact quality of life and safety. Find evidence that is used in best practice guidelines to promote continence management in people living with dementia.

4. Reflect on the need to discuss future care, including care at end of life. As these discussions ideally occur while the person still has 'capacity' to participate, what could you do to initiate such discussions?

5. How might you build on the initiatives (e.g. top 5, and the sunflower) to promote person-centred care in hospitals, residential aged care facilities and in the home setting?

A FINAL WORD

The stories of Nell, Bronwen and Melissa have provided you with different perspectives on experiences of living with dementia or caring for a person living with dementia. As you will have learnt from these stories, each person is a unique individual with, in many cases, a long and productive life in which family and friends, occupations and roles, hobbies and activities have defined who they are. In the summary to the Aged Care Royal Commission into Safety and Quality, a segment of a transcript was reported in which a husband (Mr Barrie Anderson), when asked about how to provide care for his wife, said:

It's a fairly simple message, actually, to walk in Grace's shoes, to recognise that she's had a rich past, that there's a present and that she has an evolving future (Royal Commission into Aged Care Quality and Safety, 2021).

This message applies to each individual in these stories and to all others who will need support and care from the point of diagnosis to the end of life. We hope you have acquired some valuable learning and new insights, as well as enjoyed listening to our storytellers.

CHAPTER 7

Living with stroke – the carer's perspective

Eleanor Horton

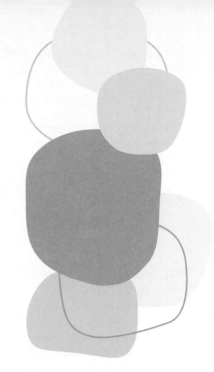

INTRODUCTION

Being a carer for someone with neurological changes is a challenge but could also be seen as an opportunity I never thought I would have. In this chapter I will try to provide you with some learning opportunities that may differ from your traditional textbook scenarios. It will be written from both the perspective of a carer and that of the registered nurse woven together. I have presented this story many times over the years, but I come back to the words from the song: 'some days are diamonds and some days are stone ... Sometimes the hard times won't leave me alone'. This is a carer's snapshot and I hope it gives you some insight into a carer's perspective. For privacy reasons, I have changed the name of the person I care for.

Before you begin

Reflect on what you may already know. Think about carers you may know – those who are in your close circle of friends or maybe the wider community. Ask yourself the following questions:
- What do you actually know about them as carers?
- What tasks does this person do as an informal carer?
- Do you know if they access any services to support their caring role?

- Do you know how they live from day to day?
- Do you know how many informal carers there are in Australia?
- Do you know how much they save the country economically?

Thirteen years on from the 2009 *Who Cares...?: Report on the inquiry into better support for carers* (House of Representatives Standing Committee on Family, Community, Housing and Youth), carers are still not recognised or embedded within reform. Provided here is a link to Carers Australia to highlight the cost associated with caring for those who remain living in their own homes (https://www.carersaustralia.com.au/caring-costs-us/).

The Value of Informal Care in 2020 Report (Deloitte Access Economics) found it would cost $77.9 billion in 2020 to care for those living within their own homes: (https://www.carersaustralia.com.au/caring-costs-us/).

What is an informal carer?

Informal care is generally defined as the unpaid care provided to older (65 years and over), dependent or disabled persons by a person with whom they have a social relationship, such as a spouse, parent, child, other relative, neighbour, friend or other non-kin (AIHW, 2021). This may involve assistance with core activities such as mobility, self-care and communication or non-core activities, such as help with household chores or other practical errands, transport to doctors or social visits, social companionship, emotional guidance or help with arranging professional care (Triantafillou et al., 2010).

In Australia the provision of informal care is primarily provided by a family member (approximately 89.8%) and mostly these are female members of the family (ABS, 2019b). Only 5% of older Australians are in residential aged care facilities, with the majority of the population choosing to stay in their home with support from carers (AIHW, 2017).

According to the Australian Bureau of Statistics (ABS, 2019a), in 2018 there were 2.65 million people (10% or 1 in 10 Australians) who provided informal care in Australia. More than one-third (35% or 929,000 people) of all carers were aged 35–54 (the average age was 50). In 2020 it is estimated that there are almost 2.8 million informal carers (Deloitte Access Economics, 2020). Approximately 1 in 11 Australians is a carer (Fig. 7.1).

The above data illustrates the steady growth of the informal carers in Australia and this needs to be considered in relation to the rise in age of carers, which is evident in the graph presented below from the report by Deloitte *The value of informal care in 2020.*

This growth is expected to continue to rise until 2030 when the report projects there will be 1.54 million informal carers.

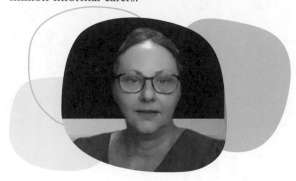

Eleanor's story

 View Eleanor's story or read the transcript.

As a nurse academic for many years I found recently that my carer responsibilities for my partner and my ageing parents were increasing, placing myself into a position where a decision was required to leave the academic world. I have been a carer for my partner for many years and through my academic connections have collaborated closely with the aged care sector and community partners. These partnerships were developed from my previous experience prior to the education field working in the aged care sector as a residential aged care facility manager and in large community organisations. With this professional life experience and knowledge, navigating the pathway of being a carer has and is a completely different experience to anything else I have experienced.

In 1947, in a small country coastal town in the South Island of New Zealand there was a first-born son called John. In February 1998 he had a quadruple coronary artery bypass graft surgery in a large city hospital. In September 1999, he decided

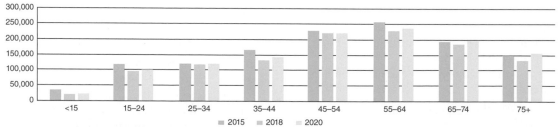

Figure 7.1 Distribution of informal carers in Australia by age, 2015 to 2020. (Source: *https://www.deloitte.com/au/en/services/economics/perspectives/value-of-informal-care-2020.html*)

to move to Australia. John gained employment at two universities and he loved life in Australia. He settled in one city about 1600 kilometres away from me. He rode a mountain bike, ran and swam. He played the guitar, piano and enjoyed singing and karaoke.

In July 2000, it was a usual night but John went somewhat early to bed as the night before had been a celebration. His flatmate woke up in the morning, saw him on the floor and presumed he was doing his exercises. But after about 10 minutes he realised there had been no movement and he didn't get a response from John. A quick call to the ambulance was actioned. Then a call to me. He didn't know first aid – I will never forget his regretful statement. I gave him instructions over the phone. Thankfully today in most states the triage operator stays on the phone and will give you help and reassurance. It's a very frightening time no matter who you are.

I was managing an aged care facility and it was the last day of our accreditation visit when I took the call just after 7.30 in the morning. Staff at the time were incredibly supportive and helpful – getting me a seat on the first flight, getting me home and packed and on the plane.

When John arrived in the Emergency Department it was very busy. His work colleagues did a roster and stayed with him, talking to him and I spoke to him via phone and they could see that he recognised my voice which was positive. This was before the days of Facetime and other tools which have changed the face of communication. As a carer, I cannot stress the importance of having difficult conversations and letting those close to you know exactly what you want to happen in an adverse event. Enduring power of attorneys and health directives are so important.

The physical pain you feel receiving the initial news of a life crisis is incomprehensible. I didn't know about young people and stroke. My experience was with the older person who often developed pneumonia and passed away or came to an aged care facility. We thought we had been through it all as he had recovered from his cardiac surgery and postoperative depression. This scenario was something completely new and out of our world. We had talked about coronary events but never stroke.

The world back then didn't have phone help lines or apps. It was a world of print and internet on a computer. A mobile phone was not a smartphone. Information wasn't easily accessible. Fast forward to today when you can access your phone and look up information about any topic. Care plans were in clinical practice but not very comprehensive and didn't include significant others. I was advised to return to work, and he would be transferred to the geriatric ward and then a nursing home. The nursing staff were very kind. They put a mattress on the floor for me and let me help with his care. I found it very frustrating as I wanted a fix and wanted him back to how he was. My background was in areas of nursing where patients' health issues could be resolved or treated but this was something where there was very minimal action. John was on bed rest, indwelling urinary catheter (IDC) and oxygen delivered via nasal prongs that continued for three days. The next day action happened – John was out to a chair and therapy began: 15 minutes of each therapy – occupational, speech and physiotherapy. I did repeat sessions of what the therapists did throughout the day. As he had not eaten and had swallowing issues, it was decided to insert a nasogastric tube on the third day. By then I was able to transfer him to a wheelchair and we frequented the seaside walkway path every day and sat in the sun. The social worker was very helpful but also very busy. I felt as if I was stuck there with very limited services. I had grown up in a small country town with very limited services but through my work experiences I knew that health services could make such a difference.

I contacted a friend who was a medical student and his advice was to move John to a large city. The hospital wouldn't enter into that conversation as he was able to be cared for where he was but it meant I could not return to work. We managed to get a private stroke specialist to accept him as a patient and he managed to secure a bed in the medical ward at a private hospital. We had to wait the two weeks to get a clearance to travel, then to arrange ambulance transfers. On reflection this was a logistical nightmare for someone outside the health system. I really had no idea. I made the decision to travel first class and risk travelling without employing someone to travel with us. John was right hemiplegic and aphasic at the time. Ummmmm, but but but, because because because – random repetitive words that meant nothing.

Fast forward to today he is still hemiplegic, mobile with an Ankle Foot Orthosis splint (AFO), uses a walking stick or power wheelchair, developed epilepsy four years post stroke, has aphasia, dyspraxia, depression, diabetes, atrial fibrillation, has a pacemaker, wears a urodome (urinary sheath) at night as he has an enlarged prostate and other general health issues.

What it feels like to be a carer

As being a carer is not a position that I applied for, or trained for or ever thought I would be, my feelings are very mixed. It's a bit like a melting pot. I had helped my grandmother care for my grandfather who had dementia and he always identified me as a nurse, but that was my limited experience as a carer. At the time of John having his first stroke I was terrified that I would not make it to him in time before another event happened as the flight was hours. There was so much that I hadn't said to him and now I might have missed the time. I recall sobbing on the plane all the way. I felt physically sick. The air steward was amazing as I was beyond being able to talk about it, but she did manage to give me some Panadol. I can't describe the mixture of feelings.

Now I have been a carer for nearly 23 years, it is a really strange role and I still don't think I do it well. I don't feel very confident at times, despite having been an academic health professional, which is completely unrelated. I really admire every carer as they appear so much more confident than I do. I asked John what kept him going when he had the stroke initially and he said it was because I was always there and I hadn't given up on him. Whenever he opened his eyes I was there.

He didn't have the brain capacity to see I was terrified, that I didn't know how to be a carer or what happened to young people when they had a stroke that took away a third of the brain. I could manage an aged care facility but here I was feeling totally inadequate with one patient. Here I was with international nursing work experiences, but I was filled with fear. Give me cardiac arrests in intensive care or theatre where I have colleagues and I have equipment. At home in the community, I am by myself and at times it is the loneliest and insecure time. When an event occurs, I press his alarm or dial 000 and that is the longest time to wait. John's epilepsy developed post stroke and atrial fibrillation has complicated our lives somewhat at times and scares me – less so now with a pacemaker. I wasn't aware of the link between brain damage and epilepsy, so it was four years post stroke before he was diagnosed. Prior to this I think he had been having absent seizures since the stroke that I attributed to delayed processing and understanding related to his aphasia. Sometimes I feel it's all too hard and I must be really thick because I cannot interpret what he is asking for and it may be something so simple. For example, what is the ensuite called when he keeps pointing to the bedroom. Charades are not my strong point. We had

a cat called Puss, which I thought would be easy for him, but after a long time I worked out when he made a continuous circle with his finger it meant the cat. Life is never static being a carer. Just when you think it is settled and there is some sense of stability, there is an upset and, until recently, being a carer who is also in full-time employment, it's just a big juggling act at times.

Comments made by other carers when I asked them about how they feel

- This all feels so hard and yet I can manage a course with thousands of students and many staff.
- I can run a business, but I don't feel capable to do this.
- At times I feel so alone in this journey.
- I am a capable person but with this experience I feel so frustrated at times.
- I am really privileged to be sharing this journey or this part of their life with them.

Things that have helped

Initially, I could not have contemplated bringing John home without knowing that he had the stamina and fortitude to continue to work at his rehabilitation. The stories of other survivors and carers at the stroke support groups we joined were supportive. It's the old story – there is always someone else who has suffered more and lost more. My parents' support was amazing and assisted me to return to work. From the beginning, post stroke, John and I agreed that rehabilitation was now his job and he could maintain the house.

He did struggle mentally for quite a while, but in those days, it was hard to access a counsellor or psychologist. Mental health services and supports are now available and encouraged if required post stroke. The aphasia, and lack of reading and writing, which had been his life, has always been a challenge. We had a variety of medication and probably it was about seven years before we had a general practitioner who understood his loss and substance abuse, and prescribed appropriate medication not just anti-depressants.

When John had the stroke, I managed to access a music therapist which was very rare in those days. She came every day and then he had a physiotherapist in the city that helped him to exercise with music for his rehabilitation. I believe music has power and throughout the years I have used it a lot to sustain me through the rough patches. Especially songs that we used to share prior to the stroke. Friends from stroke support groups and my professional friends have been invaluable along this journey. Many people say I am resilient, but I believe you are not dealt something that you can't deal with in this life, but that doesn't mean that you like it – you just get on with it. Sometimes you don't have time to think about the storms or what is actually happening, as you just get better at dancing in the rain, so they say.

Services and resources

Over the years this has been varied but the one constant in our life has been the Stroke Foundation. When I initially called them 23 years ago there were only three people and we have seen it grow phenomenally and offer so much support and so many resources to clinicians, stroke survivors and carers.

The assistive technology community has been a challenge to access, but it has grown very quickly and there are so many resources available and many are more affordable now than they were in the past. We lived in a smart home for many years, developing a platform with information technology people and researching resources that were appropriate to assist people to stay at home in the community.

The Carers' Association has always been in the background but I chose to become more involved with the Stroke Foundation, as I would like a world without stroke or at least a world without disability caused by stroke. In 2007, John ended up in resuscitation following a seizure and then it was determined that we needed more assistance for him to stay at home. It was a big decision to have carers into our home and to liaise with a community care provider! This was a big change for us to accept as I have always worked, and John was quite good with his balance and mobility. We kept up private physiotherapy and/or hydrotherapy for 14 years post stroke. Then we put in a heated pool so he could do his own hydrotherapy at home. Carers gave him different people to communicate with and sometimes it was frustrating for both of them – allowing time for him to work out what he wanted with or without words.

In 2018 John had a series of falls and the result was four stable spinal fractures, some of which may have occurred over time. He had hospital rehabilitation again followed by a transition care program and then the physiotherapy at home was increased. We had not been near a hospital for some time, so

to see the improvement in care and services was amazing. Then, in January 2021 he had a fall resulting in an intracranial haemorrhage in the same place as his previous stroke, so we were back through the whole rehabilitation journey again. This time it was so much worse for me in some ways. I think I was so shocked initially, as the older he is, the chance of not surviving becomes more real to me. The speech pathologist completed the very detailed assessment, which was a very good process. He can follow 3–4 words and this was the first time we had something concrete to help us with his speech at home. We also completed the partnership training offered online from England for aphasia and it was very good. We have always used captions on the television to assist him and he listens to audiobooks and podcasts.

That time, I had to remodel the ensuite to be a wet room and replace the carpet in the bedroom with vinyl, as when he is tired his affected leg doesn't lift as much. It is consistent change to meet his needs. Changing steps and rails to ramps for the wheelchair and shifting furniture around.

Stroke support groups have always been part of our world until recent years when the groups became challenging for him cognitively. There are many online stroke support groups now that are very helpful.

Support of health professionals

Having access to a good reliable General Practitioner and practice nurse is essential. Until recently, our practice was open seven days a week and that made such a difference to me as a working carer. Often, it is the practice nurse I need as a sounding board to tell me what to do. Or affirm for me what I am thinking as a carer, not as a nurse. Many times, I wished that I didn't have any health literacy at all. They need to be open to all alternative therapies that are available. We have tried many over the years. Not all were evidence based and perhaps the degree of helpfulness could be debated academically, but they were helpful to us at the time.

Recently, when John had a fall and had a fractured fibula – Weber B – and was in a moon boot was an extremely frustrating and upsetting time for me. In 2018 with the spinal fractures, we put in place a power wheelchair for use when he was tired or out in public. Thankfully we had the chair as with the moon boot it was so helpful and it still is as his mobility has not returned to what it was prior to the fracture. John does daily exercises and intensive hydrotherapy, but this highlighted for us both that what is a simple fracture for many is not for someone who is already differently abled.

Overall, I would like health professionals to support working carers more by offering flexible services. The pandemic has been a blessing in some ways as now we have teleheath phone and video appointments which are so much easier. Understanding aphasia and those with cognitive challenges is a skill and needs to be valued. Not all health professionals take or have the time to converse with these people. I would like to see all stroke survivors be seen by the stroke teams no matter what the cause of their admission just for continuity of care through the stroke journey.

Challenges

I suppose challenges I face are similar to those faced by many people who end up unexpectedly being a carer. Life suddenly changes without any warning. Your goals and life plans are now determined by what is realistic to include for a differently abled person. Do you keep to your plans or how far do you amend them? It's a challenge when there are so many hidden disabilities with stroke care. My partner has many of them – aphasia, dyspraxia, depression, fatigue, slight swallowing issues at times, impaired hearing on his affected side, cognitive issues, diabetes, epilepsy and of course sexual and intimacy issues. The men's health clinic was invaluable for many years with different medications (expensive) to assist him with his sexual responses and it was many years before we decided it isn't a priority for us anymore. Prior to the stroke, John was very romantic and brought me flowers and birthday surprises but all that is no longer part of him. That executive planning and thinking is different. Many parts of him as a person disappeared or were minimised with the stroke, but sometimes I get glimpses. For example, if I am very stressed at work and come home uptight, he will be playing music on YouTube to distract my thoughts. The brain is just different now.

Due to my employment, John is not entitled to a health card or concessions, and when the National Disability Insurance Scheme came in, he was then in aged care so completely missed out. The cost of his monthly medications is significant. Our focus has been his rehabilitation, including a visit to an expensive private clinic for intensive hyperbaric treatment, massage and acupuncture treatments, private physiotherapy and hydrotherapy are but some. I remained managing an aged care facility for a couple of years, but then returned to academia. I was meant to be a full-time student to complete my doctorate. Instead, it took me many years part-time to complete. Much of John's love of the European philosophers is still locked inside his head and sometimes if I was stuck on a particular idea in my research, he could go and find me a book to help me but couldn't discuss it.

Going out socially means that I usually go first and check that the place is safe and has good access to disabled toilets. So many of them focus on those people who have a left-sided disability, whereas he has a right-sided disability and needs room for a chair. Friends find it a challenge after a while when you cannot converse. For a few years, I edited and wrote presentations and took him to the philosophy conference so he could be with his old colleagues, but in the end, it was too challenging for everyone. He isn't a social butterfly and relates one-to-one to people. Luckily, we have always had great neighbours where we live that are very kind and supportive.

Mental health has always been an issue and is one that I constantly monitor for John. He has been stable for many years now and it has been such a relief. Living with atrial fibrillation is a constant anxiety-provoking issue for me – less so recently with a pacemaker. John had 21 years on Warfarin and I felt in control and as if we knew what was happening, due to frequent INR testing. The change to newer medications that require less monitoring has been helpful but sometimes improvements in practice do not suit everyone. Care needs to be individualised not standardised for all unless variations are acknowledged and valued.

The challenges are varied and many come and go. The decisions that I made, I live with. It was my choice that he would not go into an aged care facility and that cost has been high for me in many ways, but he is happy with his iPad, electric lift chair, high-back chair, over-bed trolleys, high-low bed, pressure mattress, bidet, power chair, non-slip Teva sandals, falls alarm and smart television. Not the ideal for myself or for many people, but for someone who needs high care and is still able to live in the community, it is his contentment. Relationships change throughout the stroke journey, but friendship remains and for us his rehabilitation journey continues. Life is what you make it.

Reflection

1. Reflect on any experiences that you have had with a person who is differently abled or disabled.

2. What is your knowledge of the difference between a young disabled person and an older person who is disabled?

3. Consider the difference between the National Disability Insurance Scheme and the aged care pension. If you say someone is disabled and they are over 65 years yet do not look that old, then people presume they would be covered by the NDIS. The support differences between both are considerable, so if you are providing care you need to know about the NDIS or Aged Care Services.

Inquiry

1. If you search for the carer's experience you will find that the literature is related to specific conditions and ages of development through the lifespan. Carers Australia has resources specifically related to carers, such as the report *Caring costs us: The economic impact on lifetime income and retirement savings of informal carers* (Carers Australia, 2022). They advocate and influence policy and services at a national level in Australia. Many countries will have a similar organisation to represent carers.

2. The following papers have also been selected for your consideration:
   - 'The long-term unmet needs of informal carers of stroke survivors at home: A systematic review of qualitative and quantitative studies' (Denham et al., 2022)
   - 'Informal caregiver burnout? Development of a theoretical framework to understand the impact of caregiving' (Gérain & Zech, 2019)
   - 'Caregiver burden: A concept analysis' (Zhu et al., 2020).

Action

1. Describe why it is important to understand the needs of informal caregivers in any clinical setting.

2. Review your knowledge of carer burnout and the carer burden.

3. Critically review the material listed in the Further Reading section related to care for stroke survivors and the experiences of survivors and carers and consider how this literature will inform your practice to improve care.

A FINAL WORD

There are various treatments for immediate stroke care now and innovative advances in rehabilitation so that many people may not be living a future life with multiple disabilities post stroke. **But** these options are often dependent on a set timeframe and access. Access to appropriate treatment and care for anyone who has signs or symptoms of stroke needs to be always prioritised wherever they are so they can achieve the best health outcomes.

I see the role of being an informal carer as a privilege and a choice. You are there to assist and support someone to have the best life that they can, considering all the health challenges that they are living with. The support provided by health professionals for carers to achieve the best health outcomes for the person receiving their care is immeasurable but it is always immensely appreciated. Ultimately, the goal for the best health outcome is shared by everyone.

CHAPTER 8

Living with asthma

Michelle Stubbs

INTRODUCTION

This chapter will explore two stories that provide individual perspectives – one of a healthcare professional and the other of a person living with asthma. Each story has key areas of interest that draw on the experience of the individual within a present-day Australian context and considers the issues that may impact on the person, carer, healthcare professional and the healthcare service within this milieu.

Before you begin
How our beliefs and assumptions influence practice

It's always important to ensure you are a clinician that engages in reflection. Reflection is a method of using experiential knowledge to enable professional and personal development while reinforcing continuous learning. Before viewing Zoe and Karen's stories (or reading the transcripts) take the time to reflect on the questions below and consider your knowledge about asthma and what it is like for the millions of people around the world that live with varying daily asthma symptoms. Also reflect on the aspect of living with an invisible and at times silent illness, and how people with asthma cope with this disease even though symptoms are at times not visible. Please consider your views around the below questions, and the implications that these may have on your practice.

- What do you know about asthma? Is there a cure for asthma?
- How many people are suffering from asthma globally and within Australia?
- Are Aboriginal and Torres Strait Islanders more likely to be diagnosed with asthma than non-Aboriginal Australians?
- Are there different types of asthma?
- What is it like for people to live with daily symptoms of asthma that vary in severity?
- How does this impact on one's ability to complete daily tasks like going to work, playing sport or attending university or social gatherings?
- Does living with a chronic airway disease impact mental health?
- What services or resources are you currently familiar with that people with asthma could access either online or in person?

Asthma overview

Asthma is a long-term lung condition of the airways (the passage that transports air into our lungs). Currently symptoms of asthma, including shortness of breath, chest tightness, wheeze and cough, can be managed, but there is no cure. People diagnosed with asthma have sensitive airways. When a person is exposed to 'triggers', their airways become inflamed. When the airways become inflamed, they narrow, resulting in significant persistent and troublesome symptoms. Breathing difficulties are caused by this airway narrowing and is described as breathing through a very thin tube. The narrowing of airways is known as a flare-up or asthma attack. A flare-up or asthma attack can lead to a medical emergency. A flare-up/asthma attack can develop quickly over minutes, or can gradually develop over hours, days or even weeks.

Understanding the pathophysiology, triggers, symptoms and treatment for asthma is very important when considering the experience of living with asthma. Take the time now to stop and reflect on your knowledge of asthma, including levels of disease severity, types of asthma, daily management and emergency management of asthma, and its burden and impact. Do you know what asthma triggers are? Do you know that medications for asthma now come in injectable form and not just in inhalers? Do you know the criteria healthcare clinicians use to diagnose asthma? There are many resources that can be accessed on the internet and in library resources that can help and guide you.

In the first story, Zoe discusses what it is like for people to live with asthma. She discusses specific aspects from the point of view of a person living with asthma. Symptom management, asthma control and illness limitations are highlighted. This introductory conversation provides a basis for healthcare professions to improve their levels of understanding and knowledge of the experience of living with a chronic airways disease such as asthma.

Asthma control

Asthma control is one of the main goals of asthma management. Control of asthma is achievable in most people regardless of the level of severity of their asthma. People with well-controlled asthma should be able to participate in work and school, and play sports without any limitation to breathing. 'Well-controlled asthma' means that asthma symptoms are infrequent (twice a week or less), there is no night waking due to asthma, no limitation of normal activities, and the person is at a low risk of flare-ups. 'Difficult-to-treat asthma' is when asthma symptoms remain uncontrolled (or people experience flare-ups), despite taking maximum doses of inhaled preventer medication. 'Severe asthma' is when people continue to have frequent symptoms or flare-ups (or both), despite the diagnosis having been checked, other conditions having been treated, and despite them regularly taking maximum doses of inhaled preventer medication.

Asthma and its impact (burden)

Living with asthma, and particularly severe asthma, may result in substantial burden. The main types of burden include physical, emotional and financial. Physical burden is described as the physical limitations – the inability to complete daily activities. People with severe asthma often explain how they continually struggle to breathe. Emotional burden is described as the toll asthma plays on a person's mental health. Anxiety and depression are common types of emotional burden in people with asthma. Financial burden is seen in people who are unable to work due to their asthma. Asthma medications and treatment are costly with some medications costing over $50 per month. Burden on the family, friends and loved ones of a person with asthma may also be high. Sometimes family members cannot stay employed as they are needed to care for their loved one.

Asthma first aid

An 'asthma attack' or 'flare-up' is a worsening of asthma symptoms and lung function compared with what you would usually experience day to day. An 'attack or flare-up' may come quickly or over a few days and may lead to an asthma emergency. Asthma first aid is first-line management of an 'attack or flare-up'. Asthma first aid should be commenced if a person suddenly has difficulty breathing, is unable to speak in full sentences, is coughing, wheezing, or has a feeling of chest tightness.

Asthma resources and services

Over past years, improvements have been made in the provision of resources for people with all types of asthma. There are numerous apps that can be downloaded on phones and other devices to monitor asthma symptoms. Asthma-related telehealth services and severe asthma clinics are increasing in locations around Australia. Resources and services, however, are only useful if people who need them know about their existence.

Severe asthma is debilitating, but there is hope

Living with severe asthma is debilitating; however, advances in management and treatments give people hope. Common treatments include preventers and relievers. Preventers contain anti-inflammatory medications (corticosteroids) and are usually inhaled daily. Relievers such as salbutamol give fast relief from narrowing airways and are used when a person experiences a flare-up. New injectable medications are now available to people with severe asthma. These medications are called biologics. Biologic medications have fewer side effects and can be self-administered. A treatment that does not involve medication for severe asthma is bronchial thermoplasty. This is a procedure which involves passing a scope into the lungs where heat waves are delivered to reduce the amount of muscle in the airways, which have thickened due to successive flare-ups. This procedure helps make breathing easier.

Living well with severe asthma

There are many things that people living with severe asthma can undertake to help relieve symptoms and disease burden. These include participating in education sessions with their treating clinician, using a written asthma action plan, actively monitoring symptoms and engaging in physical activity. Activities that promote mindfulness (for example, yoga and meditation) may also increase wellbeing in people with severe asthma.

Interpersonal skills are important

Healthcare professionals may be considered by people with severe asthma to be the most important people in healthcare. It is critical that nurses possess capable interpersonal skills to establish positive relationships with patients, their carers, families or loved ones and other healthcare professionals. Active listening is considered perhaps the most interpersonal skill of them all. Active listening is a learned skill for effective communication. It involves complete attention to what a person is saying, listening carefully while showing interest, and not interrupting. It requires awareness of the content, intent and feeling of the person speaking. Some people with severe asthma may first and foremost want their treating clinicians to listen and pay attention to what they are actually saying, they want to be 'heard'. Other interpersonal skills include concise verbal communication, patience and awareness, the ability to build relationships, conflict resolution and critical thinking.

Self-advocacy in people with severe asthma

In general, self-advocacy is the ability to speak up for yourself. Self-advocacy in healthcare may be seen as taking an active role in managing one's health. In severe asthma, self-advocacy involves learning about severe asthma, asthma control and the numerous treatment options available so that decisions can be made about management that are right for an individual. Resilience is also as important as self-advocacy. Resilience in chronic illness is often thought to be a process of effectively adapting to maintain or regain emotional wellbeing. It is often a process through which a person's thoughts and behaviours overcome distress and optimise positive outcomes.

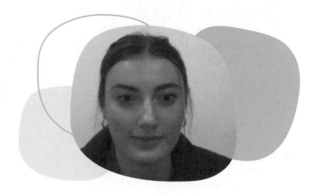

Zoe's story

 View Zoe's story or read her transcript.

Zoe Sacmaroski is a 20-year-old undergraduate teaching student who was diagnosed with asthma as a child. Zoe describes her experience of living with asthma for many years, detailing her symptoms, asthma control and challenges faced with living with asthma, as well as useful resources in asthma management.

Reflection

1. What are the components of asthma control?
2. How do you know when asthma is well controlled versus not well controlled?
3. What is the most frequently used questionnaire to measure asthma control?
4. How often do you think a person with asthma should have their level of asthma control assessed by a healthcare professional?
5. What is it like to live with asthma?
6. To what extent are family members/loved ones and friends affected by someone's asthma?
7. Do people with asthma feel like a burden to others?
8. What are the most common injectable medications administered to people diagnosed with severe asthma?
9. Do you know the common medications (inhalers only) used in asthma management? Can you list eight classifications of inhalers?
10. What medications are safe to use to treat asthma during pregnancy?
11. Do you think asthma is a serious medical condition?
12. Does the chance of an asthma attack make people with asthma scared to be alone?
13. Does a person with asthma have increased anxiety or fear if they do not have a puffer on hand?
14. If a common symptom for a person with asthma is a cough, would COVID-19 increase or worsen the cough?
15. If a person with asthma does test positive for COVID-19, should they increase their usual asthma medications?
16. Is an asthma flare-up more dangerous when a person is COVID-19 positive?
17. What are effective ways information could be disseminated to people with asthma?
18. Does the provision of telehealth services in rural/remote areas result in better asthma control?
19. What are the barriers to telehealth services for people with asthma?
20. Do specialist asthma clinics exist in every state and territory of Australia?
21. Does being under the care of an asthma specialist improve asthma outcomes?
22. In rural Australia, how do people with asthma access emergency services?
23. What agencies in Australia are researching and leading the way in asthma management and treatment advances?

Inquiry

1. Asthma Australia is a for-purpose, consumer organisation with a history of improving the lives of people with asthma. Asthma Australia's mission is 'To help people to breathe so they can live freely'. Asthma Australia operates across New South Wales, Victoria, Queensland, Tasmania, South Australia and the Australian Capital Territory and works in partnership with the Asthma Foundations of Western Australia and the Northern Territory to deliver evidence-based prevention and health strategies to more than half a million people each year. Asthma Australia offers training and education for schools and workplaces, resources and also has products available for purchase to manage asthma symptoms. A varied range of information is available from Asthma Australia whose vision is to have a community free of asthma.

2. The National Asthma Council Australia are the national authority for asthma knowledge, setting the standard for asthma care. The National Asthma Council provides information about understanding asthma, living with asthma and asthma first aid for both community members and healthcare professionals. The National Asthma Council is a collaboration of four member bodies: (i) Australasian Society of Clinical Immunology and Allergy; (ii) Australian Primary Health Care Nurses Association; (iii) The Pharmaceutical Society of Australia; and (iv) The Royal Australian College of General Practitioners. A sizable amount of information can be found on the National Asthma Council's website, including the Asthma Handbook.

3. As an adjunct to this, you may wish to review what steps should be taken during a flare-up or attack. It should be noted that quick action may help prevent an asthma attack from becoming an asthma emergency. Signs of an asthma emergency include severe shortness of breath, major issues with speaking, blue-coloured lips (called cyanosis) or little or no relief from inhaler use.

4. The mission statement of Asthma WA is 'Leading the education and empowerment of Western Australians to take control of their respiratory health'. Asthma WA is a registered charity delivering education and support for people with asthma and those around them. Asthma WA provides an assortment of education and advice mediums, including telephone, face-to-face clinics, video conferencing (telehealth) and online resources and education packages. Education and support through Asthma WA is easily accessible.

5. The following papers have also been selected for your consideration:

   • 'Patients with severe uncontrolled asthma: Perception of asthma control and its management' (George et al., 2022)

   • 'Factors affecting quality of life and asthma control in older adults with asthma' (Schuckmann, 2022)

   • 'Asthma in adults' (Nanda & Wasan, 2020)

   • 'Health-related quality of life burden in severe asthma' (McDonald et al., 2018)

   • '"It's like being on a roller coaster": The burden of caring for people with severe asthma' (Majellano et al., 2021)

   • ' "… I've said I wish I was dead, you'd be better off without me": A systematic review of people's experiences of living with severe asthma' (Eassey et al., 2019)

   • 'A shift in asthma treatment according to new guidelines: An evaluation of asthma patients' attitudes towards treatment change' (Holst et al., 2023)

   • 'Management of life-threatening asthma: Severe asthma series' (Garner et al., 2022).

7. Review the paper titled 'Management of Life-Threatening Asthma: Severe Asthma Series' by Garner and colleagues (2022). Develop a flowchart outlining the journey from the Emergency Department to the Intensive Care Unit.

8. Are family members the 'forgotten people' in asthma management?

9. Did the mental health of people with asthma decline during the COVID-19 pandemic?

10. Critically review current literature on telehealth services. Consider both the enablers of and barriers to telehealth services in people with asthma.

11. Review available literature publicly available online relating to asthma services and support. Is the literature easily accessible? Would an ageing asthma population be able to access such information?

12. Determine additional ways or avenues in which asthma information could be distributed. How would people with asthma benefit from additional information being easily accessible?

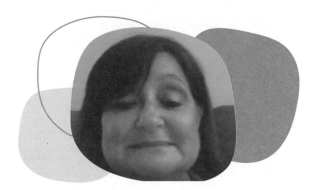

Action

1. Describe the impacts of living with asthma.

2. Review your understanding of symptom management, asthma control, public perception and daily limitations of living with asthma.

3. How is well-controlled asthma defined?

4. What role do triggers play in managing asthma symptoms?

5. What are commonly prescribed asthma inhalers?

6. How does regular review of asthma symptoms improve the lives of people living with asthma?

Karen's story

 View Karen's story or read her transcript.

Karen Johnson is an individual who was diagnosed with severe asthma at the age of 19 years. Karen discusses her journey through life living with asthma, highlighting the burden and impacts of living with severe asthma and the value of healthcare professionals. Karen also emphasises the importance of self-advocacy and knowledge in living with chronic illness.

Reflection

1. Do you think symptoms of asthma worsen as the day progresses? Or do people with severe asthma wake up with uncontrolled symptoms?

2. What are the impacts of extended hospitalisations due to asthma?

3. Contemplate Karen's words: *I've lost most of the last ten years of my life*. How do people cope with feeling like they have lost years of their life due to asthma?

4. What do you know about pulmonary rehabilitation, focused breathing techniques and bronchial thermoplasty for the treatment of severe asthma?

5. Is the physical impact of severe asthma worse than the psychological impact of living with severe asthma?

6. What are current treatment guidelines for severe asthma?

7. How many people per year visit emergency departments for asthma flare-ups in Australia?

8. Does a positive or negative attitude influence asthma control?

9. Can you describe how people identify with chronic illness?

10. What is the difference between calling yourself an asthmatic and saying you have asthma?

11. Do you know if there is an association between overall physical health and asthma control?

12. Are levels of activity reduced in people with severe asthma compared with those with mild to moderate asthma?

13. What are the benefits of a well-informed and educated person living with severe asthma?

14. What are the key features of self-management?

15. How do people with severe asthma maintain resilience?

16. How common is anxiety and depression in people with asthma versus those with severe asthma?

17. What are the long-term consequences of ignoring the burden of living with severe asthma?

18. Think about when a clinician only observes a patient. What important cues about their illness may be overlooked? Can patients look better than they feel?

19. Patient satisfaction is one of the most important factors in determining the success of healthcare service delivery. How does active listening increase patient satisfaction?

20. What behaviours demonstrate that a healthcare professional is listening?

21. Complete the following:
    - I believe the most important skill a healthcare professional needs is …
    - To me, communication is …

22. What issues may arise when a person with severe asthma lacks self-advocacy?

23. List important areas of asthma education. Do you believe education about self-monitoring of asthma symptoms to be most significant?

24. Consider the importance of perseverance when living with severe asthma. Could it be implied that perseverance is a key attribute in coping with severe asthma?

25. Think about what is involved in growing resilience. What role can family members, significant others and healthcare professionals play in developing resilience in people living with severe asthma?

26. Complete the following:
    - I believe self-advocacy leads to …
    - Resilience is importance because …

Inquiry

1. The Centre of Excellence in Severe Asthma (funded by the National Health and Medical Research Council) developed the Severe Asthma Toolkit to address an identified gap in the availability of severe asthma education resources for clinicians. This Severe Asthma Toolkit provides tools to help clinicians provide optimal care for people with severe asthma and is targeted at clinicians in primary and specialist care, in both private and public clinic settings. The Centre of Excellence in Severe Asthma brings together researchers from across Australia. The centre is working to develop innovative approaches to understand why severe asthma occurs, developing tools and programmes to improve disease management and improving access to new therapies.

2. Another resource providing information on severe asthma is Healthtalk Australia. Healthtalk Australia is a collaboration of researchers from the Royal Melbourne Institute of Technology

(officially RMIT University), the University of Sydney, Monash University and the University of New South Wales. Healthtalk Australia conducts research into the experiences of health and illness. Healthtalk Australia aims to contribute to the development of the qualitative research knowledge base about people's experiences of health and illness (including carers' experiences and health professionals' perspectives), and use the results to create public online resources targeting the Australian community, researchers, health professionals and policymakers. The Healthtalk Australia website is used to: (i) support patients, carers, family members and friends; (ii) provide clinical education and professional development; (iii) promote quality improvement/experience-based health service co-design; and (iv) develop policy and clinical guidelines. You may wish to visit the Healthtalk Australia website and familiarise yourself with the information it provides.

3. The Global Initiative for Asthma (GINA) was launched in 1993 in collaboration with the National Heart, Lung, and Blood Institute, National Institutes of Health, USA, and the World Health Organization. GINA works alongside healthcare professionals, patient representatives, and public health officials around the world to reduce asthma prevalence, morbidity and mortality. In 2022, GINA released a report noting that difficulties exist in distinguishing symptoms of anxiety and depression from asthma symptoms (GINA, 2022). This may therefore lead to misdiagnosis. Misdiagnosis is problematic in people with severe asthma. If you are unfamiliar with features of misdiagnosis in severe asthma, you may wish to explore the latest GINA report available from their website. You will also find helpful information on anxiety and depression, and when referral to psychiatrists should occur.

4. The Australian College of Nursing (ACN) is an Australian professional nursing organisation that advocates at state and federal levels with Ministers and Health Departments to provide valuable insight and recommendations from a nursing perspective. The ACN is also the Australian member of the International Council of Nurses (ICN) and advocates for the profession at both a national and an international level. The ACN website is a publicly available and useful site for nurses looking for information relating to current nursing initiatives, education and national nursing events.

5. The Severe Asthma Toolkit has already been introduced earlier in this chapter; however, now is a good time to revisit the website and further explore particular components of severe asthma management and to also watch additional stories of the experience of living with severe asthma. Commonly, people with severe asthma talk about the burden of disease and the challenges of day-to-day living. As severe asthma is a complex disease, there is no one-size-fits-all approach to management. You may wish to revisit the Severe Asthma Toolkit at this stage and review information under the 'management', 'living with severe asthma' and 'resources' tabs: https://toolkit.severeasthma.org.au/

6. The following papers have also been selected for your consideration:

   • '"Nothing about us without us"— What matters to patients with severe asthma?' (McDonald et al., 2022)

   • 'The experience of living with severe asthma, depression and anxiety: A qualitative art-based study' (Stubbs et al., 2021)

   • 'Principles for nursing practice: Persistent asthma' (Allen, 2022)

   • 'Living well with severe asthma' (Stubbs et al., 2019)

   • 'Treatment strategies for asthma: Reshaping the concept of asthma management' (Papi et al., 2020)

   • 'A feasibility randomised controlled trial of Novel Activity Management in severe ASthma-Tailored Exercise (NAMASTE): Yoga and mindfulness' (Hiles et al., 2021)

   • 'Using a knowledge translation framework to identify health care professionals' perceived barriers and enablers for personalised severe asthma care' (Majellano et al., 2022)

   • 'Interpersonal communication in healthcare' (Chichirez & Purcărea, 2018)

   • 'Importance of teamwork communication in nursing practice' (Alkhaqani, 2022)

   • 'Teaching self-advocacy skills: A review and call for research' (Schena et al., 2022)

   • 'Patient advocacy: An antidote to loneliness and more' (Walker, 2022)

   • 'The effect of patient self-advocacy on patient satisfaction: Exploring self-compassion as a mediator' (Salazar, 2018).

Action

1. Describe the burden of living with severe asthma. Does burden differ between mild to moderate asthma and severe asthma?

2. Describe the impacts asthma places on family members and significant others.

3. Compare how common symptoms of anxiety and depression are in people with severe asthma to people with non-severe asthma.

4. What is the impact of anxiety and depression?

5. How are symptoms of anxiety and depression assessed in people with asthma?

6. Consider the five elements of active listening.

7. Review the strategies that enhance active listening skills.

8. Is there one particular element of active listening that you need to work on?

9. Critically review current literature in relation to self-advocacy and resilience.

10. Write a list of questions that a person with severe asthma can ask their healthcare professional that helps them to understand their own needs.

11. Identify and list characteristics of resilience.

12. Determine ways in which levels of resilience can be increased.

A FINAL WORD

As a healthcare professional it is vital to understand that asthma is a heterogeneous, complex and common chronic respiratory disease. While the majority of people with asthma can be treated effectively with currently available medications, a proportion of people cannot. These people remain a challenge from treating clinicians and are often diagnosed with severe asthma. One must remember there is no 'one size fits all approach' to asthma management. People with severe asthma face a consistently heavy burden with daily symptoms such as coughing and shortness of breath, and frequent asthma attacks often requiring hospitalisation. To better assist people with severe asthma, nurses should take the time to actively listen and understand their concerns. This helps in being prepared to address issues as they arise, resulting in better asthma outcomes. The stories of both Zoe and Karen have provided you with a brief 'snapshot' of their experiences and understanding of asthma, with a deeper look at severe asthma. We hope you have enjoyed the experience!

CHAPTER 9

Living with cardiac disease

Ritin Fernandez

INTRODUCTION

This chapter will explore caring for people with cardiac illness from the perspective of a nurse, two patients and a carer. All four participants will provide their experiences of working or living with heart disease, within the context of contemporary Australian health and social care services. The aim is to explore the views of the patients and carers as well as the health professionals and their perception of the challenges faced by people who are living with cardiac illness.

Before you begin

Chronic cardiac disease includes a variety of conditions that affect the heart. These include:

- blood vessel disease, such as coronary artery disease
- abnormal heart rates (arrhythmias)
- disease of the heart muscle
- issues with the heart valves.

Based on self-reported data from the Australian Bureau of Statistics 2020–21 National Health Survey, an estimated 571,000 Australians aged 18 and over (2.9% of the adult population) had coronary heart disease (CHD) (Australian Bureau of Statistics, 2022). In 2020, an estimated 56,700 people aged 25 and over had an acute cardiac event in the form of a heart attack or unstable angina equating to approximately 155 events each day. Twelve per cent of these cardiac events were fatal.

How our beliefs and assumptions influence practice

Clinicians need to use their reflective and reflexive thinking skills in clinical practice. While reflection focuses on your thoughts, feelings and actions, reflexivity involves being aware of your preconceived ideas and beliefs and noticing patterns in your experience about illness and patients. Cardiac disease is a common chronic illness and some of you might have experience caring for a family member or friend with the illness. These experiences could be positive or negative, resulting in the development of preconceived ideas about the illness and the health services. It is important, therefore, to be aware of our biases and learn from our experiences.

Before viewing the recordings, or reading the transcripts from Lois, Sharon, Nicholas and Heather, please consider your views on the following questions and the implications that these might have on your care.

- What is your opinion of people living with chronic heart disease?
- Have you or any family member suffered from some form of heart disease?
- Has your experience changed your perception of cardiac disease?
- What are your beliefs about who can get the disease?

Heart disease: A brief clarification of concepts and terms

Coronary heart disease is a condition that involves reduced or lack of blood supply to the heart muscle due to narrowing or complete blockage of a coronary artery. The blockage is caused due to a build-up of fatty substances in the coronary arteries. There is no one cause of coronary heart disease, but certain risk factors can increase the chance of developing the condition. These risk factors are classified into modifiable and non-modifiable risk factors. The modifiable risk factors include smoking, excessive alcohol consumption, lack of exercise, stress and being overweight or obese. The non-modifiable risk factors include family history, age, being male and ethnicity. Some diseases such as high cholesterol, high blood pressure, diabetes and depression can also increase the risk of developing coronary heart disease (Khoja et al., 2023; Zhang et al., 2023). Coronary heart disease develops over time.

While some people experience symptoms of coronary heart disease, others may not. Many people find out that they have coronary heart disease when they experience chest pain or have a myocardial infarction also called a heart attack. Symptoms of heart attacks include chest pain, pain in the neck, jaw, left arm, shoulder, upper back or abdomen (stomach), a feeling of being cold and sweaty, shortness of breath, fatigue, nausea or vomiting, light-headedness or dizziness, and heart palpitations. The symptoms vary between different people, and especially between males and females. For example, men are more likely to have chest pain while women are more likely to have other symptoms such as shortness of breath, nausea and extreme fatigue (Haider et al., 2020).

Arrhythmia, also called irregular heartbeats, is a problem that occurs when the rate or rhythm of the heartbeat is not normal. For example, the heart rate may be too fast (tachyarrhythmia) or too slow (bradyarrhythmia), or not regular. Factors that can cause arrhythmia include having had a heart attack, smoking, congenital heart defects and stress. The prevalence of arrhythmias in the general population ranges between 1.5% and 5% with atrial fibrillation the most common arrhythmia, affecting 2% to 9% of people (Desai & Hajouli, 2022). Arrhythmias can be treated with medication or procedures to control the irregular rhythms.

Cardiomyopathy is a disease of the heart muscle. In this condition, the heart is unable to pump blood to the rest of the body and can lead to heart failure. Heart failure affects about 1% to 2% of people in Australia. The signs and symptoms of heart failure include shortness of breath or trouble breathing, fatigue, swelling in the ankles, feet, legs and abdomen, dizziness, fainting and arrhythmias (Al-Omary, 2021). Over time, cardiomyopathy gets worse; however, treatment helps to slow the progression and improve the patient's quality of life.

Heart valve disease includes the malfunctioning of one or more of the valves in the heart causing the blood circulation to be disrupted. Heart valve disease affects nearly 2% of Australians. The signs and symptoms of heart valve disease include abnormal sound when listening with a stethoscope (heart murmur), chest pain, fainting, dizziness or light-headedness, irregular heartbeat, palpitations, shortness of breath, swelling of ankles and feet and tiredness. Heart valve disease can require surgery to repair or replace the heart valve (Aluru et al., 2022).

Some added context

- Cardiac rehabilitation is a multifaceted evidence-based intervention that provides benefits to patients with any form of heart disease or heart failure, and promotes health-related quality of life. Cardiac rehabilitation is led by health professionals and involves personalised support, exercise and education to strengthen the heart. Cardiac rehabilitation usually starts in the hospital and continues in the outpatient clinics after discharge for up to three months, depending on the type of program offered. Cardiac rehabilitation helps the individual make long-term lifestyle changes to live a longer, healthier life. It helps in the recovery after a heart event, procedure or the diagnosis of a heart condition. Participation in cardiac rehabilitation is associated with a 32% lower risk of all-cause mortality compared with non-participation (Akpinar & Oral, 2023; Dibben et al., 2023).
- **Coronary Angiogram** is a procedure where a dye is injected and is visible by an x-ray

machine as it travels through the blood vessels of the heart. The x-ray machine then rapidly takes a series of images (angiograms). The results of the procedure provide evidence if there is a restriction in blood flow going to the heart (Curtis et al., 2020).

- **Percutaneous Coronary Intervention** (PCI): Previously known as angioplasty with stent, PCI is a non-surgical procedure that uses a thin flexible tube to place a stent in the blood vessel that is narrowed due to atherosclerosis. Opening the blood vessel that is narrowed improves blood flow, thereby decreasing or relieving chest pain (Curtis et al., 2020).

- **Coronary artery bypass graft surgery** (CABG) is a surgical procedure used to bypass the blocked portion of the coronary artery with a portion from another healthy blood vessel. The blood vessels used for the graft may be a piece of vein from the leg or an artery from the chest or wrist. One end of the blood vessel is attached above and the other end is attached below the blockage thus enabling reperfusion to the heart muscle. CABG is an invasive procedure and is usually performed under general anaesthesia. Patients normally stay for approximately seven days in the hospital following CABG to ensure proper recovery.

- Coronary heart disease is the leading cause of death in women in the United States. In Australia, CHD is the second highest cause of death in women after dementia. On average in Australia, 20 women die each day due to coronary heart disease, which equates to one death almost every hour of every day. Heart disease in women can occur at any age, but as they grow older the risks change (Australian Institute of Health and Welfare, 2019). The evidence suggests that when compared with men, women are much less likely to undergo treatment for a heart attack or angina. In addition, attendance at cardiac rehabilitation and adherence to medications is poor among women. They are also less likely to make heart-healthy lifestyle changes.

- Living with a cardiac disease affects not only the individual diagnosed with the illness but also their families and carers.

- **Carers** are people who look after and help with the day-to-day living of their family member or friend. Carers provide unpaid care and support to people with a chronic condition, disability, mental illness, terminal illness, an alcohol or other drug issue or who are frail or aged. In Australia, carers are an integral part of the health system with approximately 10% of the people listed as carers. More than 70% of all carers are middle-aged females (ABS, 2018).

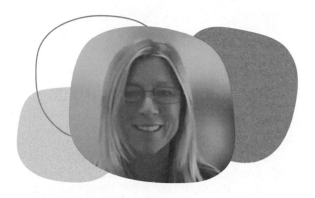

Lois's story

 View Lois's story or read her transcript.

Lois Mantell is a Registered Nurse providing cardiac rehabilitation services to people discharged from two large regional hospitals in the Central Coast Local Health District of NSW. Lois talks about her experience of providing cardiac rehabilitation services for people with heart disease. Lois shares her perspective as a Registered Nurse, reflecting upon the clinical and personal challenges arising when providing cardiac rehabilitation services. She also shares her perception of challenges faced by her client group, and potential solutions to enhance care and improve service user outcomes.

Reflection

1. What in your opinion is the role of the cardiac rehabilitation services?

2. Should cardiac rehabilitation be provided only after a patient is discharged?

3. What are some of the factors that impact the provision of cardiac rehabilitation services?

4. In your opinion, what is the role of the cardiac rehabilitation nurse in providing care for people with cardiac illness?

5. After watching the video, you might also want to reflect again on your assumptions about cardiac disease. Also, consider how it might feel to attend cardiac rehabilitation as a person with heart disease.

Inquiry

1. The Australian Cardiovascular Health and Rehabilitation Association (ACRA) is the peak body that provides support and advocacy for multidisciplinary health professionals to deliver evidence-based best practices across the continuum of cardiovascular care. The aim is to empower health professionals to achieve optimal and equitable outcomes for all affected by cardiovascular disease: https://www.acra.net.au/

2. The Heart Foundation is the trusted peak body working to improve heart disease prevention, detection and support for all Australians. The mission of the Heart Foundation is to 'reduce heart disease and improve the heart health and quality of life of all Australians through our work in risk reduction, support, care and research': https://www.heartfoundation.org.au/

3. The following papers have also been selected for your consideration:

   • 'A new era in cardiac rehabilitation delivery: Research gaps, questions, strategies, and priorities' (Beatty et al., 2023)

   • 'Exercise-based cardiac rehabilitation for coronary heart disease: A meta-analysis' (Dibben et al., 2023)

   • 'Cardiac rehabilitation in women, challenges and opportunities' (Sawan et al., 2022)

   • 'Safety of home-based cardiac rehabilitation: A systematic review' (Stefanakis et al., 2022).

Action

1. Explain why it is important to understand the needs of people living with cardiac disease.

2. Review your knowledge of the role of cardiac rehabilitation nurses in providing comprehensive care to people with cardiac disease.

3. Critically review the four above papers relating to cardiac rehabilitation. Consider how this literature might inform your practice given that cardiac rehabilitation is an evidence-based intervention for people with cardiac illness.

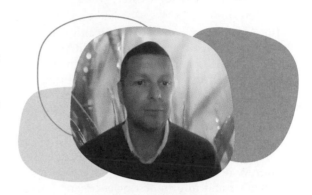

Nicholas's story

 View Nicholas's story or read his transcript.

Nicholas Jago is a 42-year-old gentleman with two children who lives in NSW. Nick works for a large company and has the opportunity to work from home. Nick loves soccer and coaches his children in the sport. Nick shares his experience of being diagnosed with heart disease and how it has impacted his life. Nick also shares his experiences of how he overcame these challenges.

Reflection

1. What could be some of the reasons why Nicholas was diagnosed with cardiac disease?

2. How would you make younger people aware of cardiac disease?

3. Why do you think young people develop cardiac disease?

4. What could be some of the physical, social, emotional and financial consequences for young people with heart disease?

5. You might also want to critically reflect upon your own beliefs and assumptions about young people developing coronary heart disease. Do you or a relative have any experience of having a PCI or CABG?

Inquiry

1. The full pathway to cardiac recovery can be accessed and reviewed here: https://www.heartfoundation.org.au/getmedia/c77bac1d-4de5-4000-8e4c-0ecb1365f1b2/A_Pathway_to_Phase_II_Cardiac_Recovery_(Full_Resource).pdf

2. The Australian Cardiovascular Health and Rehabilitation Association Inc. (ACRA) has developed 10 quality indicators and the data collected contributes to regular monitoring and reporting of the quality and delivery of cardiac rehabilitation across Australia. The quality indicators for cardiac rehabilitation support healthcare providers to: identify barriers and enablers to increase referrals, improve delivery processes, improve patient outcomes and inform best practices and alternative models of care.

3. The following papers have also been selected for your consideration.

    • 'Preprocedural anxiety in the transradial cardiac catheterization era' (Fernandez et al., 2021)

    • 'Predictors of cardiovascular complications in patients with chronic ischemic heart disease after bypass surgery' (Akhmedov & Narziev, 2023)

    • 'Operative outcomes of women undergoing coronary artery bypass surgery in the US, 2011 to 2020' (Gaudino et al., 2023)

    • 'Sex difference in outcomes of acute myocardial infarction in young patients' (Sawano et al., 2023).

Action

1. Describe why it is important to understand the emotional needs of people undergoing procedures for heart disease.

2. Critically review the above papers relating to PCI and CABG. Consider how this literature might inform your practice and how cardiac nurses can provide evidence-based care to people with coronary heart disease.

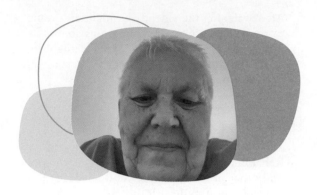

Sharon's story

 View Sharon's story or read her transcript.

Sharon Kennedy is a 75-year-old lady living in regional NSW and loves to travel around the globe. Sharon has been to countries in every continent including spending eight days in Antarctica. Sharon shares her experiences with her diagnosis of heart disease and her ways of living with the chronic condition.

Reflection

1. How can you as a cardiac nurse help women cope with living with heart disease?

2. What do you think are some of the issues contributing to the growing number of women having coronary heart disease in Australia?

3. What actions can you take to raise awareness about heart disease in women?

4. Why do you think heart disease in Australian women is currently under-recognised, under-diagnosed and under-researched?

5. You might also want to critically reflect upon your own beliefs and assumptions about women and heart disease by asking yourself the following questions.

    • I believe that heart disease is for men, and cancer is a real threat to women.

    • I always assume that heart disease doesn't affect women who are fit and exercise regularly.

Inquiry

The following papers have also been selected for your consideration:

- 'Delays to hospital presentation in women and men with ST-segment elevation myocardial infarction: A multi-center analysis of patients hospitalized in New York City' (Weininger et al., 2022)
- 'Mechanisms of coronary ischemia in women' (Huang et al., 2022)
- 'Trends in inequities in the treatment of and outcomes for women and minorities with myocardial infarction' (Montoy et al., 2022)
- 'Sex differences in cardiac rehabilitation outcomes' (Smith et al., 2022).

Action

1. Describe some of the emotional and mental challenges faced by women living with coronary heart disease.
2. Briefly research the women-specific services available in your area so that women can improve their lifestyle and reduce their risks of heart disease.

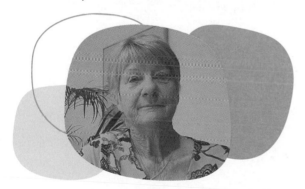

Heather's story

 View Heather's story or read her transcript.

Heather Sykes is 75 years old, retired and living in Sydney, NSW. Heather shares her experiences as a carer, looking after her husband who was diagnosed with heart disease and heart failure. Heather speaks about some of the practical, financial and human challenges faced by carers when looking after a person with cardiac illness.

Reflection

1. What are the key skills needed for a carer looking after a person with cardiac disease?
2. What do you think are the effects of caring on the carer's physical, social, mental and financial wellbeing?
3. Why do you think that there is a growing number of carers in Australia?
4. How do you think carers can be supported when looking after people with cardiac disease?
5. You might also want to critically reflect upon your own beliefs about carers, e.g. 'I believe that you're only a carer if the person is your family member and lives with you' or 'I always assume that carers are in good health themselves'.

Inquiry

The following papers have also been selected for your consideration.

- 'Experiences of family caregivers in caring for patients with heart failure at Jakaya Kikwete Cardiac Institute, Dar es Salaam, Tanzania: A qualitative study (Mcharo et al., 2023)
- 'A systematic review comparing cardiovascular disease among informal carers and non-carers' (Lambrias et al., 2023)
- 'Attachment insecurities, caregiver burden, and psychological distress among partners of patients with heart disease' (Laflamme et al., 2022).

Action

1. Describe some of the emotional and mental challenges faced by carers when caring for a person with cardiac disease.
2. Briefly research the support services available in your area for carers.
3. Heather spoke about the financial support she received from the Department of Veterans' Affairs. How do you think carers who don't receive this service manage?

A FINAL WORD

Technical and pharmacological innovations have reduced the incidence of CHD mortality and morbidity; however, it remains the leading cause of mortality globally. CHD affects people irrespective of gender, age, ethnicity and educational level. The associated costs resulting from the physical and psychosocial disabilities place a significant burden on the patients, their families and the community. Evidence suggests that programs providing risk-factor education and counselling with or without supervised exercise are effective in promoting cardiac health and enabling the individual to live with the condition. Carers play a major role in improving the quality of life of those living with heart disease.

The stories indicate the challenges faced by health professionals as they strive to provide evidence-based care to patients. The stories from the patients and carers also demonstrate the consequences of living with cardiac disease. It is therefore vital that nurses understand these challenges to provide empathetic evidence-based care to improve the wellbeing of patients and their carers.

CHAPTER 10

Living with chronic kidney disease

Ginger Chu

INTRODUCTION

This chapter will explore patients' experience of living with chronic kidney disease and clinicians' experience of caring for patients with kidney disease. Chronic kidney disease (CKD) is a growing public health issue responsible for a substantial burden of illness and premature death. People living with CKD often experience high burdens due to the disease and the associated treatments.

The aim of this chapter is to explore the challenges people with kidney disease face. A patient and three clinicians were invited to share their experiences. A patient spoke about his experiences and personal challenges of living with CKD, followed by a multidisciplinary team (a renal physician, a renal nurse practitioner and a renal social worker); each spoke about their experiences of caring for people with kidney disease. This inclusion of a patient and a multidisciplinary team would provide an overview of patient care within a contemporary Australian health system and how each health professional collaborates and communicates together to address the complex needs of the patient.

Before you begin
How our beliefs and assumptions influence practice

It's always important for clinicians to be reflexive. This involves being aware of your preconceived assumptions, biases and beliefs about a particular disease and how this might influence your practice. For example, some people believe that kidney disease only affects older people or assume that poor lifestyle choices are always the cause of kidney disease. The misconception can lead to blame and judgement towards people with kidney disease. By understanding and addressing these beliefs and assumptions, healthcare professionals can help people with kidney disease manage their illnesses more effectively and improve their quality of life. Before viewing the recording or reading the transcripts from Dave, Carla, Sarah and Thida, please consider your views on the following questions and the implications that these might have on your practice.

- What is your opinion of people with kidney disease?

- Have you, or any family member, suffered from kidney disease or required dialysis?

- Consider what it might be like living with kidney disease and having to attend a dialysis centre three days a week to receive treatments. How would this affect your life or your family's life?

- What are your beliefs about people who have kidney disease?

- Do you know anyone who suffers from kidney disease? How do they manage their kidney disease?

- What services or resources are you currently familiar with that would be useful to support people with kidney disease?

Chronic kidney disease and dialysis: A brief clarification of concepts and terms

Chronic kidney disease refers to a condition characterised by a gradual loss of kidney function over time (Webster et al., 2017). There are five stages to kidney disease based on the severity of kidney function loss. Stages one and two are often recognised as the early stage of kidney disease, and when the kidney function deteriorates to stage three or four, that is when most people are likely to experience symptoms and be diagnosed with kidney disease. Unfortunately, some individuals' kidney disease can lead to kidney failure, often seen in stage four or five of kidney disease, which can be life-threatening if kidney replacement therapy such as dialysis or kidney transplant is not started.

Dialysis is a kidney replacement therapy that removes waste and excess fluid from the blood when the kidneys stop working (Sargent & Gotch, 1996). There are two different types of dialysis: peritoneal dialysis and haemodialysis. Both dialyses would require a patient to go through a surgical procedure to make an 'access' for dialysis treatment. With haemodialysis, a machine removes blood from the patient's vascular access (fistula or catheters), filters it through an artificial kidney and returns the cleaned blood to the patient. This procedure normally takes place in a hospital or a dialysis centre over three to four times a week.

Some added contexts

- **Fistula:** An arteriovenous (AV) fistula connects an artery and vein to create a large vein that makes it easier to access the bloodstream for dialysis purposes (Wasse & Beathard, 2019). However, an AV fistula takes time to mature before it can be used for dialysis. If a person requires dialysis

urgently, a catheter (thin tube) may be inserted into a person's neck, chest or leg as short-term access. There is a much higher risk of infection associated with catheters. Therefore, a fistula is often recommended for people who require long-term dialysis. If kidney disease is detected early and monitored regularly, there should be adequate time to discuss it with the patient and prepare them for suitable vascular access.

- **Renal diet and fluids:** The most identified challenge by patients with CKD is diet and fluid restriction. When a person's kidneys become less effective at removing unwanted fluid and waste, it is important to reduce the waste and fluid build-up by controlling what they eat and drink in between dialysis sessions. Certain food, due to the high level of potassium or phosphate, can accumulate waste too quickly in between dialysis sessions. Therefore, planning a balanced diet becomes crucial. Restricting fluid intake is considered the toughest part of all by patients as dialysis only replaces a part of the kidney function and is only typically performed 4–5 hours a day, 3–4 times a week. Dialysis patients need to limit their fluid intake to avoid fluid overload, which can cause symptoms such as shortness of breath and oedema. This can be a challenging task for patients when they are thirsty or during a hot day. A renal dietitian can help patients find ways to manage thirst and plan for a healthy diet based on an individual's unique situation.

- **'Feeling drained and lethargic':** Dave mentions 'feeling drained and lethargic' after dialysis. This is a common side effect of haemodialysis treatment. Other common side effects of haemodialysis such as a drop in blood pressure, muscle cramps, headache and nausea or vomiting, altogether can affect a person's daily activity, social life and overall quality of life. Dave spoke about how these symptoms can impact a person getting in and out of dialysis. He also spoke about how these symptoms may be mitigated by good fluid and diet control.

- **Renal social worker:** Living with kidney disease may affect many aspects of a person's life. Besides the stress and worry about physical illness, the person and their carers or families may also be concerned about finances, future plans, as well as a range of emotions relating to health and changes to lifestyles. Starting dialysis is a major life change for people with kidney disease. Patients may experience emotional repercussions due to changes in body imaging, treatment-related fatigue or loss of independence. In addition, the restrictions to diet and fluids and the lack of freedom to travel, as Dave mentioned in his story, can all take a toll on a person's emotional wellbeing. Renal social workers provide services such as counselling, grief and loss support, information and referral to appropriate services and are, therefore, an integral part of a multidisciplinary team.

- **Pre-dialysis education:** When a person's kidney disease deteriorates and they are no longer able to adequately remove excess waste and fluids in the body, they will require kidney replacement therapy to sustain life. Currently, the main kidney replacement therapy options are: transplant, haemodialysis at home, haemodialysis in the hospital or community centre, peritoneal dialysis or conservative care. Each option has different advantages and disadvantages and impacts on patients' lives. It is important that the patient and their carers or families understand the requirement of each treatment so they can make an informed decision. Pre-dialysis education is designed to help patients and their caregivers to understand the treatment options and provide support to improve their quality of life.

- **Shared decision making:** As Carla mentioned, it is important that clinicians support patients by ensuring there is a shared decision-making process. Shared decision making is defined as 'an approach where clinicians and patients make decisions together using the best available evidence' (Elwyn et al., 2010). As mentioned above, due to the different impact that each kidney replacement therapy option has on a person's life, patients and their carers need to be able to make an informed decision to choose the best treatment for themselves. During the shared decision-making process, clinicians share their professional knowledge with the patient, and, in turn, patients share their personal views on their life and how each treatment fits into their lifestyle. Collaboratively, a decision should be made between the patient and the clinician regarding the best treatment for the patient.

- **Nurse practitioner:** Nurse practitioner is an advanced nursing role that works autonomously using their extended scope of practice to make recommendations for medications, treatment and onward referrals to other specialists (NMBA, 2021). The role of the nephrology nurse practitioner in Australia ranges from managing

patients in the early stages of CKD (stage 1–3), where the focus is on slowing the progression to kidney failure, through to those receiving kidney replacement therapy or those requiring conservative care (Bonner et al., 2022).

- **'Silent Killer':** Chronic kidney disease is often referred to as a 'silent killer' because a person could potentially lose up to 90% of kidney functions before symptoms present (de Zeeuw, 2008). In Australia, one in three adults has an increased risk of developing kidney disease (Kidney Health Australia, 2023). Understanding the cause of kidney disease and early detection are the keys to preventing and slowing down kidney disease progression.

- **Symptom burdens:** Patients with chronic kidney disease experience high symptom burdens, similar to patients with cancer (Sepúlveda et al., 2002). The common symptoms reported by patients, such as fatigue, sleep disorders, pruritus and nausea/vomiting can contribute to reduced quality of life (Fletcher et al., 2022). Understanding the burden of symptoms can be used as the basis for treatment choices and for identifying care priorities, which are likely to improve the quality of care and patients' quality of life.

- **Timing of dialysis:** When is the best time to start long-term dialysis in patients with chronic kidney disease remains unclear. Renal physicians like Thida have the ultimate responsibility to discuss this with the patient and their family to ensure there is a balance between mortality and the burden of a substantially longer period spent on dialysis. As Thida mentioned, the decision regarding when to dialyse patients, what dialysis modality and how to ensure patients and carers understand and are involved in a shared decision-making process is a daily challenge for renal physicians.

- **Kidney transplant:** A kidney transplant is an operation to place a healthy, functional kidney that was donated by a person to a person whose kidneys are no longer working. Kidney transplantation is considered an alternative to long-term dialysis. However, not every patient with chronic kidney disease is eligible or able to receive a donor kidney. In Australia, a person can wait between five and seven years for a suitable kidney once they become eligible (Transplant Australia, 2023). The steps required for patients to become eligible transplant recipients can be lengthy and exhausting.

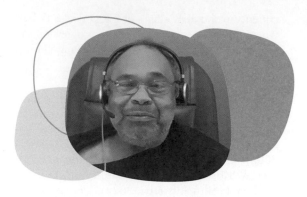

Dave's story

 View Dave's story or read his transcript.

David Beale is a 50-year-old Indigenous person who is currently undergoing three days a week haemodialysis treatment due to advanced kidney disease. David talks about his experience of living with kidney disease and the impact of haemodialysis treatment on his personal life. He also talks about the challenges of accessing dialysis treatment for people who live in rural and remote areas of Australia from the perspective of Indigenous people. Finally, he shares some of his personal thoughts on what healthcare professionals can do to enhance care and support for people with kidney disease.

Reflection

1. What is your understanding of kidney disease?
2. Can you list the challenges identified by Dave? Can you think of any more to add to the list that he has not identified? In your opinion, what would be the greatest challenge? And why?
3. Can haemodialysis replace normal kidney function?
4. What do you think if people say everyone has equal access to dialysis service if they require it?
5. After watching the video, you might also want to reflect on your own assumptions about

kidney disease. Also, consider how it might feel to attend dialysis as a person living with chronic kidney disease.

Inquiry

1. National Kidney Foundation (NKF) is an organisation that supports kidney patients and families by raising awareness about the danger of kidney disease. There is a wide range of information developed by NKF on issues related to kidney disease, especially dialysis and transplant. At this point you might like to take the time to access the website and search for 'treatment & support' to identify the specific needs of people with kidney disease undergoing dialysis: https://www.kidney.org/
2. The following book chapter and papers have also been selected for your consideration.
3. 'Principles for nursing practice: Chronic kidney disease', Chapter 22 of *Living with chronic illness and disability: Principles for nursing practice*, 4th ed. (Bonner & Brown, 2022)
4. 'Arteriovenous vascular access-related procedural burden among incident hemodialysis patients in the United States' (Woodside et al., 2021)
5. 'Experiences and perspectives of dietary management among patients on hemodialysis: An interview study' (Stevenson et al., 2018)
6. 'Prevalence and risk factors of postdialysis fatigue in patients under maintenance hemodialysis: A systematic review and meta-analysis' (You et al., 2022).

Action

1. Describe why it is important to understand the needs of people living with kidney disease undergoing dialysis treatment.
2. Review your understanding of the common challenges faced by people with kidney disease undergoing dialysis treatment.
3. Critically review the three above papers relating to burdens associated with dialysis treatment. Consider how this literature might inform your practice.

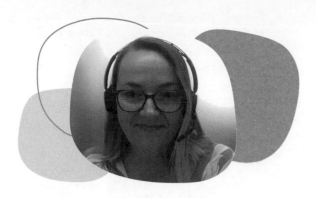

Carla's story

 View Carla's story or read her transcript.

Carla Silva is a senior renal social worker working in a community dialysis centre in regional Australia. In her role as a renal social worker, she provides care for people in different stages of kidney disease (from diagnosis to treatments when kidney function deteriorates). Carla speaks about the common challenges that people with kidney disease face and the available support and resources for people living with kidney disease.

Reflection

1. What are the key skills needed for a renal social worker?
2. What role do renal social workers provide in the provision of care for people with kidney disease?
3. Do you think the role of the social worker is important in a multidisciplinary team? If so, why?
4. Do you think pre-dialysis education is important to people with kidney disease? What may be the impact of pre-dialysis education on patient outcomes?
5. Reflect on your current practice. Do you foster opportunities for shared decision making in your care delivery?
6. You might also want to critically reflect upon your own beliefs and assumptions about the importance of emotional support in healthcare services. Do you or a relative have any experience in providing or receiving such care?

Inquiry

1. The Nursing and Midwifery Board of Australia (NMBA) regulates the practice of nursing and midwifery in Australia by developing professional standards of practice for all comprehensively registered nurses. The decision-making framework developed by NMBA states:

   'The primary motivation for any decision about a care activity is to meet people's health needs or to enhance health outcomes. The decision about activities should be made in partnership with the person, supporting **shared decision-making**'.

   • NMBA decision-making framework for nursing and midwifery can be accessed and reviewed here: https://www.nursingmidwiferyboard.gov.au/codes-guidelines-statements/frameworks.aspx.

2. The following papers have also been selected for your consideration.
   • 'The role of the nephrology social worker in optimizing treatment outcomes for end-stage renal disease patients' (Callahan, 2011)
   • 'Multidisciplinary predialysis education reduced the inpatient and total medical costs of the first 6 months of dialysis in incident hemodialysis patients' (Yu et al., 2014)
   • 'Asking the right questions: Towards a person-centered conception of shared decision-making regarding treatment of advanced chronic kidney disease in older patients' (Verberne et al., 2022).

Action

1. Describe why it is important to understand the emotional needs of people living with kidney disease in any clinical setting.
2. Review your knowledge of the role of renal social workers and how they can work collaboratively with other members of the kidney multidisciplinary team in hospitals and dialysis centres.
3. Critically review the three papers above and consider how each member of the kidney multidisciplinary team contributes to shared decision making to improve patient outcomes.

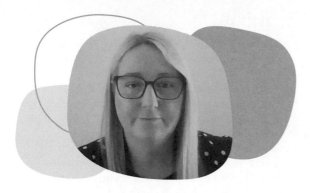

Sarah's story

 View Sarah's story or read her transcript.

Sarah Russo is a clinical nurse practitioner who works in a large tertiary referral hospital in regional New South Wales, Australia. The nephrology service in this hospital includes a 16-bed inpatient ward, an in-centre dialysis unit and five community dialysis units. Sarah speaks about the role of nursing in caring for people with kidney disease, the common challenges people living with kidney disease face and what nursing care can be provided to support patients through these challenges.

Reflection

1. What are the key skills needed for a nephrology nurse practitioner working with patients with kidney disease?

2. What do you think about the kidney disease burden in the Australian health system?

3. What are some issues that affect renal patients' quality of life?

4. What can be done to prevent kidney disease or slow the progression of kidney disease?

5. You might also want to critically reflect upon your own beliefs and assumptions about chronic kidney disease by asking yourself the following questions.

- How do I know that my family or I are not at risk of developing chronic kidney disease?
- Does every patient with chronic kidney disease require dialysis treatment?

Inquiry

1. The nurse practitioner has an extended scope of practice that is different from that of a registered nurse. The Nursing and Midwifery Board of Australia (NMBA) regulates this advanced practice by developing professional standards for nurse practitioners. NMBA nurse practitioner standards can be accessed and reviewed here: https://www.nursingmidwiferyboard.gov.au/Codes-Guidelines-Statements/Professional-standards/nurse-practitioner-standards-of-practice.aspx

2. The following papers have also been selected for your consideration.

- 'The impact of the advanced practice nursing role on quality of care, clinical outcomes, patient satisfaction, and cost in the emergency and critical care settings: A systematic review' (Woo et al., 2017)
- 'Renal disease: A common and a silent killer' (de Zeeuw, 2008)
- 'Symptom burden and health-related quality of life in chronic kidney disease: A global systematic review and meta-analysis' (Fletcher at al., 2022).

Action

1. Describe some of the physical, emotional and mental challenges that might be faced by a person with chronic kidney disease.

2. Sarah mentioned a couple of symptoms that are commonly experienced by patients with chronic kidney disease – can you please outline more symptoms?

3. Sarah spoke about chronic kidney disease being a 'silent killer'. Critically review the paper suggested above and consider how this might inform your practice.

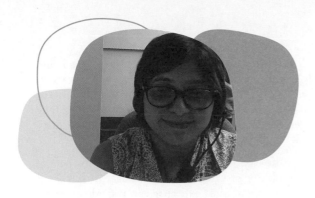

Thida's story

 View Thida's story or read her transcript.

Thida Myint is a senior staff specialist in nephrology and kidney transplant. In her role as a physician, she provides continuous care for patients while they are in hospital or when discharged to an ambulatory setting. Thida talks about the challenges she faces as a physician caring for people with kidney disease.

Reflection

1. What decisions does a person with advanced kidney disease need to make when their kidney functions deteriorate?

2. Is kidney transplant the optimal medical treatment for advanced kidney disease?

3. What might patients' experiences be while waiting for a transplant or when having fears about rejection?

4. You might also want to critically reflect upon your own beliefs and assumptions about kidney transplant by asking yourself the following questions.

    • Does every patient with advanced kidney disease have an equal opportunity for treatment modality?

    • Does a kidney transplant provide a better quality of life for patients with advanced kidney disease compared with other treatment modalities?

Inquiry

1. Transplant Australia is an organisation that supports kidney transplant recipients, donors and their families by raising awareness about organ donation. There is a wide range of information on this website to support patients and their families while either on a waiting list, living with donors or post-transplant on topics related to kidney transplants. At this point you might like to take the time to access the website and search for 'living with your transplant' to understand the specific needs of people living with kidney transplant: https://transplant.org.au/

2. The following papers have also been selected for your consideration.

    • 'Balancing everyday life – Patients' experiences before, during and four months after kidney transplantation' (Nielsen et al., 2019)

    • 'Life and expectations post-kidney transplant: A qualitative analysis of patient responses' (Tucker et al., 2019)

    • 'Timing of dialysis initiation to reduce mortality and cardiovascular events in advanced chronic kidney disease: Nationwide cohort study' (Fu et al., 2021).

Action

1. Describe some of the physical, emotional and mental challenges that might be faced by a person waiting for a kidney transplant.

2. Thida mentioned there are a few tests required of patients as a pre-screening for the eligibility for a kidney transplant. Can you please outline some of these?

3. Critically review the papers suggested above and consider how patient experiences might inform your practice.

A FINAL WORD

Chronic kidney disease (CKD) is a prevalent health condition worldwide; however, it can lead to a number of serious health consequences, particularly if it progresses to end-stage kidney disease when renal replacement therapy is required to sustain life. CKD is more common in certain populations, such as older adults, people with hypertension or diabetes and those with a family history of kidney disease. Early detection and management can prevent or delay the progression of chronic kidney disease.

All healthcare professionals form an important part of the multidisciplinary team to care for people with CKD. Our patient's story has illustrated the complexity of CKD and the impact of CKD on people's life. A team of healthcare professionals with different areas of expertise can provide comprehensive care for people with CKD, address their physical, social and emotional needs and improve overall quality of life.

CHAPTER 11
Living with diabetes

Jane Frost

INTRODUCTION

This chapter will explore the experience of people living with diabetes from the perspective of three individuals. Each person will discuss diabetes care from their own perspective and/or lived experience.

Before you begin
How our beliefs and assumptions influence practice

Clinicians need to be aware of their own knowledge, skills and attitudes towards health conditions. In this chapter we will explore diabetes in its different forms, what it is like to care for people living with diabetes and what people who have lived with diabetes for many years would like you to know. Before you start, please reflect on your own knowledge, skills and attitudes in relation to diabetes by considering the following questions.

- Can you easily describe the different types of diabetes?

- Do you know what treatments are available?

- What is your opinion of people with diabetes?

- Do you know anyone who lives with diabetes in any form?

- Consider if your own experience or interaction has influenced your view of diabetes.

- Have you heard of the chronic care model of care?

Different types of diabetes
Type 1 diabetes

Diabetes Australia defines Type 1 diabetes as an auto-immune condition where the body's own immune system is activated to destroy the beta cells in the pancreas, which produce insulin. We do not know what causes this autoimmune reaction; however, environmental factors are thought to set off the process. Type 1 diabetes is not linked to modifiable lifestyle factors. Currently there is no cure and it is lifelong.

Type 1 diabetes:
- occurs when the pancreas does not produce insulin

- represents around 10 per cent of all cases of diabetes and is one of the most common chronic childhood conditions

- in children, usually has an abrupt onset and the symptoms are obvious
- in adults, has a slower onset
- symptoms can include excessive thirst and urination, unexplained weight loss, weakness and fatigue and blurred vision
- is managed with insulin injections several times a day or the use of an insulin pump.

Type 2 diabetes

Diabetes Australia defines Type 2 diabetes as a condition in which the body becomes resistant to the normal effects of insulin and gradually loses the capacity to produce enough insulin in the pancreas. The condition has strong genetic and family-related (non-modifiable) risk factors and is also often associated with modifiable lifestyle risk factors. We do not know the exact genetic causes of type 2 diabetes. People may be able to significantly slow or even stop the progression of the condition through changes to diet and increasing the amount of physical activity they do.

Type 2 diabetes:

- is diagnosed when blood glucose levels are high due to insulin produced by the pancreas not working effectively and/or the cells of the body do not respond to insulin effectively (known as insulin resistance), over time the condition progresses and the pancreas does not produce enough insulin (reduced insulin production)
- represents 85–90 per cent of all cases of diabetes
- usually develops in adults over the age of 45 years but is increasingly occurring in younger age groups including children, adolescents and young adults
- is more likely in people with a family history of type 2 diabetes or from particular ethnic backgrounds
- may first present as a complication of diabetes such as a heart attack, vision problems or a wound that does not heal well
- is managed with a combination of regular physical activity, healthy eating and weight reduction. As type 2 diabetes can be progressive, many people will need oral medications and/or insulin injections in addition to lifestyle changes over time.

Diabetes in pregnancy

Diabetes in pregnancy can occur through pre-existing disease, i.e. those already diagnosed with either type 1 diabetes or type 2 diabetes or through gestational diabetes (defined below).

Gestational diabetes

Diabetes Australia defines gestational diabetes mellitus (sometimes referred to as GDM) as a type of diabetes that occurs during pregnancy. Women with gestational diabetes can still have a healthy baby but it is important that gestational diabetes is managed to reduce the risk of developing complications during pregnancy. Gestational diabetes will not lead to your baby being born with diabetes; however, it can increase the risk of your baby developing type 2 diabetes later in life. Gestational diabetes is diagnosed when higher than normal blood glucose levels first appear during pregnancy. Most women with gestational diabetes will no longer have diabetes after the baby is born. However, some women will continue to have high blood glucose levels after delivery. Gestational diabetes is the fastest growing type of diabetes in Australia, affecting thousands of pregnant women. Between five and 10 per cent of pregnant women will develop gestational diabetes. All pregnant women should be tested for gestational diabetes at 24–28 weeks of pregnancy (except those women who already have diabetes). Women who have risk factors for gestational diabetes should be tested earlier in their pregnancy.

Concepts to consider

- **Changes in diabetes care (knowledge):** Rebecca talks about advances in care and describes her journey from glass syringes to an insulin pump. What do you know about recent advances in diabetes care, such as continuous glucose monitoring and insulin pumps? People with diabetes will present in all areas of health care, so what do you need to know about the different types of diabetes to provide safe effective care?
- **Listening (skills):** Rebecca talks about the key skill of listening to the patient. In chronic conditions patients often know more about their illness than the health professional does. They live with diabetes 24 hours a day, 7 days a week. Reflect on this in terms of your practice and/or your observation of practice.
- **Stigma (attitudes):** Rebecca talks about stigma and feeling judged. She also talks about being called a junkie as a child and dealing with body issues as a teenager. Had you considered these aspects of living with diabetes?

- **A nursing role in diabetes (knowledge):** Ruth mentioned her role as Clinical Nurse Consultant in diabetes, there are many other roles such as Diabetes Nurse Practitioner and Diabetes educator, but it is important to recognise that understanding the care required for a person living with diabetes is important even if it is not your speciality.

- **Chronic care model (skills and attitudes):** Ruth mentioned the chronic care model as opposed to an acute care model. Reflect on your understanding of each, noting that literature has been provided for you to review. This is a recognised way of caring for people with chronic illness.

- **Awareness (knowledge):** Jane discussed awareness of diabetes and common misconceptions and its impact on the person living with diabetes. Reflect on how misconceptions may impact the nurse–patient relationship.

- **Partnering with consumers (skills):** The National Safety and Quality Health Service Standards defines 'partnering with consumers'. How does this relate to the care of people living with diabetes?

- **Perceptions (attitudes) and the concept of being different (knowledge):** Understanding the psychosocial aspects of diabetes is important as it may lead to patients making decisions about treatment that results in sub-optimal outcomes.

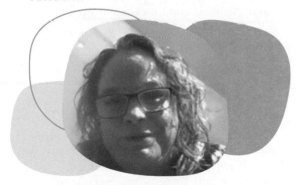

Rebecca's story

 View Rebecca's story or read her transcript.

Rebecca Hutchison is a person living with diabetes and an insulin pump educator.

Reflection

After watching the video, you might also want to reflect again on your own knowledge skills and attitudes about diabetes.

Inquiry

The following papers have also been selected for your consideration.

- 'Insulin pumps: From inception to the present and toward the future' (Alsaleh et al., 2010)
- 'Stigma in people with type 1 or type 2 diabetes' (Liu et al., 2017)
- *Diabetes: Australian facts* (AIHW, 2023)
- 'Insulin pump therapy' (Nimri et al., 2020).

Action

1. Describe why it is important to understand the treatment options for people living with diabetes.
2. Review your knowledge of the physical, psychological and social impact of a **diagnosis** of different types of diabetes.
3. Consider how you can better prepare yourself for caring for a person living with diabetes.

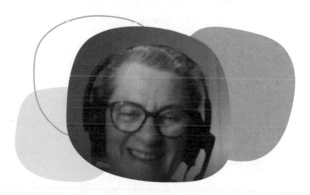

Ruth's story

 View Ruth's story or read her transcript.

Ruth Pollard is a Diabetes Clinical Nurse Consultant (CNC) for a territory-wide endocrinology service.

Reflection

1. Consider the potential differences in approach when caring for a patient with a chronic condition.

2. What are the key skills needed for health professionals who work with people living with diabetes?

3. What are the career opportunities for nurses in caring for people living with diabetes?

4. You might also want to critically reflect upon your own beliefs and assumptions about the importance of partnering with patients.

Inquiry

1. The NMBA *Registered Nurse standards of practice* can be accessed and reviewed here: https://www.nursingmidwiferyboard.gov.au/codes-guidelines-statements/professional-standards/registered-nurse-standards-for-practice.aspx

2. Focus on standard 2 and reflect on standard 2.3 and 2.7 and consider how these elements are important for diabetes care and reflected in the videos:

    • 2.3 'recognises that people are the experts in the experience of their life'

    • 2.7 'actively fosters a culture of safety and learning that includes engaging with health professionals and others, to share knowledge and practice that supports person-centred care'.

3. The following documents/papers have also been selected for your consideration.

    • National diabetes nurse education framework 2020–2022 (NDSS, 2020)

    • National Safety and Quality Health Service Standards (Australian Commission on Safety and Quality in Health Care, 2021)

    • 'Effectiveness of chronic care models: Opportunities for improving healthcare practice and health outcomes: A systematic review' (Davy et al., 2015)

    • National Strategic framework for chronic conditions (Department of Health and Aged Care, 2020).

Action

1. Describe why it is important to understand the needs of people living with diabetes in any clinical setting and reflect on standard 2 of the NMBA *Registered nurse standards for practice*.

2. Review your knowledge of the *National Strategic Framework for Chronic Conditions*.

3. Consider how the health strategies and literature provided might inform your practice.

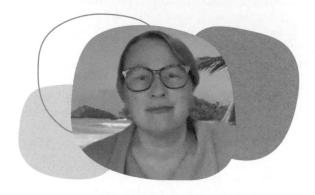

Jane's story

 View Jane's story or read her transcript.

Jane Frost is a person living with diabetes and a nurse, nurse academic and educator.

Reflection

1. Had you previously thought about the impact on diabetes in terms of someone's life apart from the medication they might need?

2. What could you do to improve care you give to people living with diabetes?

3. What misconceptions did you have about diabetes?

4. What do you think when you hear someone described as non-compliant?

5. Critically reflect upon how your knowledge, skills and attitudes have changed and what you have learnt about diabetes as different conditions and about people living with diabetes.

Inquiry

The following papers have also been selected for your consideration.

• 'Enablers and barriers to effective diabetes self-management: A multi-national investigation' (Adu et al., 2019)

- *Australian diabetes strategy 2021–2030* (Department of Health and Aged Care, 2021)
- 'Women's experiences of a diagnosis of gestational diabetes mellitus: A systematic review' (Craig et al., 2020)
- 'Assessing the impact of diabetes on quality of life: What have the past 25 years taught us?' (Speight et al., 2020).

Action

1. Describe the key priorities of the Australian National Diabetes Strategy.
2. Briefly research the services available for someone living with diabetes in your area.
3. Consider the literature provided above about people's experiences of diabetes and consider how you could affect/influence change.

A FINAL WORD

Diabetes is often seen as a single diagnosis but in fact there are several types that are treated differently because the underlying pathophysiology is different. A diagnosis of diabetes can be life changing particularly for young people diagnosed with type 1. However, a diagnosis of type 2 diabetes can be equally challenging because of the stigma and sometimes guilt involved. The key thing to remember is that diabetes affects the whole person and impacts physical, mental and social aspects of their life. Working to enable individuals living with diabetes to cope, manage and understand their illness is important, and a fundamental role of nurses working in endocrinology clinics.

CHAPTER 12

Living with chronic disease – breast cancer

Cannas Kwok

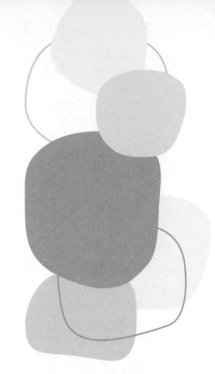

INTRODUCTION

This chapter will explore the experiences of breast cancer from the perspectives of a woman who has finished her cancer treatment and from a healthcare professional (physiotherapist) who looks after women living with breast cancer. Different from other chronic diseases, cancer is often seen as a frightening disease because being diagnosed with cancer is often linked to a death sentence. The challenges faced and encountered by survivors of breast cancer may be unique to that cohort.

While a woman living with breast cancer will be interviewed to share her experience with breast cancer through the journey from being diagnosed, going through the treatment and living with it, the physiotherapist will talk about her experiences in providing supportive care to women living with breast cancer. The aim is to provide a better understanding about the challenges of living with and experiencing this chronic disease from the perspectives of both patients and healthcare professionals, with the secondary aim of improving supportive care and promoting quality of life of cancer survivors.

Before you begin

Cancer is the second leading cause of death globally, after heart disease. In Australia, the incidence rates for cancer overall have been rising steadily over the past 20 years. Given the advanced technology in early detection and improvements in treatment, numbers of cancer survivors have increased significantly. Cancer survivor is defined as 'a person from the time of diagnosis onwards' (Cancer Council, 2023b). Many survivors require long-term care; therefore, providing quality care for cancer survivors

has become one of the key priorities in healthcare services.

While cancer treatment could be physically traumatising, the experiences of cancer extend beyond the physical domain. The psycho-social and emotional impact of cancer can be lifelong and unforgettable. 'Survivorship care' is a popular term used in cancer care that refers to follow-up care, once primary cancer treatment is finished. It includes managing treatment side effects and psychological and emotional needs as a result of diagnosis and treatment. In order to deliver patient-centred care, understanding patents' experiences both physically and psychologically, and displaying empathy will remain important considerations for healthcare professionals to bear in mind.

- Compared with other chronic diseases, what do you think about the challenges that are unique to cancer patients?
- Have any of your family members, relatives or friends ever been diagnosed with cancer?
- What do you think about the impact a loved one's cancer diagnosis may have on the family?
- What do you think about the psychological and social impact of cancer that women living with breast cancer may experience?
- What resources and services do you think are important to support the survivorship care for cancer survivors?

Challenges for women with breast cancer

Although prostate cancer has overtaken breast cancer for the first time and was the most diagnosed cancer in Australia in 2022, breast cancer remains the most common cancer among women in Australia and globally. Being diagnosed with any cancer type typically results in a range of emotions, but being diagnosed with breast cancer can be even worse because of the psychological effects of surgery on an organ representing femininity. In addition, the physical and psychological impacts of the diagnosis and treatment remain even after treatment. For instance, physical impacts can include hair loss and chronic fatigue, both of which may result in body image impairment. They can also impact financial security due to inability to maintain employment, while meeting the additional costs involved with cancer treatment. Not surprisingly, worry about cancer recurrence is one of the most common psychological impacts. Before viewing Linda's story, who went through breast cancer treatment some time ago, please reflect upon the questions below and consider what challenges women with breast cancer face throughout the cancer journey. As a healthcare professional, think about what resources and support could be included in survivorship care to promote quality of life for women with breast cancer.

- What do you think about the challenges that women face when they receive a breast cancer diagnosis?
- What do you think about the challenges they face during treatment?

- What services or support in the community do you know that are available to support breast cancer survivors and their families?

Challenges of follow-up with specialist and communication

Existing evidence identifies two major factors that have significant impact on clinical health outcomes. As already discussed, one of those factors is patient experience; the other is communication. One of the issues that Linda shared during her follow-up appointment with the specialist was the communication skills of the specialist. Reflect on your own clinical practice.

- What do you think about your communication skills with patients?
- What are effective communication skills that can be applied in clinical practice?
- How does the communication between health professionals and patients affect patients' satisfaction?
- Why are communication skills important as a healthcare professional?

Informational and social support needs

It is well known that both information and social support are vital components in achieving a high quality of life for cancer patients. Linda speaks about her disappointment when attending an information session conducted by a nurse about the side effects of chemotherapy. In addition, she shared her experiences of feeling lonely during the cancer journey due to lack of social support. Based on your experience as a healthcare professional:

- what kind of information do you think the cancer patients need the most and why?
- what is the role of information support for cancer patients/survivors and their families?
- what is the role of social support for cancer patients?
- why is a support group so important for cancer patients/survivors?
- what was Linda's suggestion in terms of specific social support for breast cancer patients?
- do you know of any cancer support groups in your community?

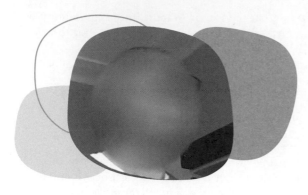

Linda's story

 View Linda's story or read her transcript.

Linda Heaton, a 65-year-old lady, was diagnosed with breast cancer three years ago. Linda has received surgery and chemotherapy treatment. She shares her experiences and the challenges she faced living with cancer.

Reflection

Treatment for cancer may involve chemotherapy, surgery and radiotherapy. These therapies are invasive and have the potential to result in long-lasting and significant side effects, including hair loss and weight gain. There is also the possibility of removal of one or both breasts which can result in body image impairment, a psychological distress that women with breast cancer are more likely to encounter. Linda has shared her experiences in this regard during the interview. Take a moment to thoroughly think about her experiences and answer the following questions.

1. What are the side effects Linda was experiencing as a result of her cancer treatment?

2. How have these side effects impacted on her physically and psychologically?

3. How have her experiences changed your perception of women living with breast cancer?

4. What are the roles of healthcare professionals in supporting women with breast cancer through their cancer journey and in their survivorship?

5. How does understanding the experiences of breast cancer patients change your perceptions of their needs? How does it impact on your future practice as a healthcare professional?

6. Describe how culture may impact on breast cancer experiences among women from minority cultures. What are the implications for healthcare professionals?

7. What kind of support and resources are essential for supporting women living with breast cancer?

Inquiry

After reviewing the video of Linda's story, are her experiences similar to what you thought about women with breast cancer? Linda has discussed a number of challenges she faced in her cancer journey and made some suggestions about how these challenges could be addressed. Could you identify what they are by addressing the following questions?

1. What was her first reaction to the cancer diagnosis?

2. Why was she angry?

3. What was the long-term psychological impact of having a cancer diagnosis?

4. How did the COVID-19 pandemic impact on her cancer journey and access to social support?

5. What are the challenges she encountered during cancer treatment?

6. Do you think the current healthcare services have met the needs of women with breast cancer?

7. What was her suggestion in terms of specific social support for breast cancer patients?

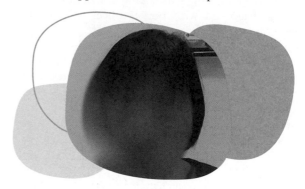

Joey's story

 View Joey's story or read her transcript.

Dr Joey Smith, an experienced physiotherapist who specialises in managing lymphoedema for women living with breast cancer, works in a cancer care centre located in a teaching hospital. Joey has been working in the position for more than 20 years. Her role is managing lymphoedema for women with breast cancer, from the pre-operative stage through to survivorship.

Lymphoedema, one of the most common side effects of breast cancer treatment, is swelling due to blockage of, damage to or removal of lymph nodes as a result of cancer treatment. Consequently, the level of movement of the affected arm will be restricted. Recent data suggest that more than 70 per cent of breast cancer patients developed lymphoedema within the first year after surgical treatment. Lymphoedema is a chronic condition that requires daily and long-term management. In addition to the physical impact, such as heaviness of limb and pain, some breast cancer survivors experience psychological distress through this constant reminder of their cancer diagnosis and treatment. Given its high prevalence and severe impact on breast cancer patients physically and psychologically, providing care and support for breast cancer survivors with lymphoedema is an essential factor in promoting their quality of life.

Joey, an experienced physiotherapist with expertise in lymphoedema management, discusses some of her challenges in providing care for women with breast cancer. The challenges have been categorised into three main areas: patients, organisational, and healthcare professional (physiotherapist). In terms of organisational challenges, resources have been mainly focusing on treatment. Managing lymphoedema, as a side effect of treatment, is not a priority. From the patients' perspective, attention has been fully occupied with frequent medical appointments and recovery after the cancer treatment. Women living with breast cancer are not aware of the importance of preventative health, to prevent developing lymphoedema. As a physiotherapist looking after breast cancer patients with lymphoedema, the major challenge is the fact that working in breast cancer care is quite an uncommon area of physiotherapy.

Reflection

1. What are the top five health priority areas in Australia?

2. Compared with other chronic diseases, is cancer care one of the priority areas for resources in the current healthcare system? Why?

Inquiry

1. In our current healthcare system, what are the challenges to optimising care for women with breast cancer who have developed lymphoedema?

2. From the patients' perspective, what are the challenges for management of lymphoedema?

3. From the physiotherapist's perspective, what are the challenges to providing care for breast cancer survivors with lymphoedema?

4. In your clinical experiences, what challenges have you encountered while looking after women with breast cancer?

Action

In this final section of the chapter, you will take some time to reflect on what you have learnt and how the learning impacts on your practices for supporting breast cancer survivors. Revisit the stories shared by Linda and Joey, the further reading provided and the websites for supportive cancer care and survivorship care plan, then answer the following questions to consolidate your learning about looking after women with breast cancer.

'The term supportive care refers to services that help cancer patients, their caregivers and their families to cope with the disease and its treatment throughout the patient's pathway and to help the patient maximising treatment benefits in order to cope in the best possible way with the effects of the disease' (Cancer Australia, 2023a).

1. Describe why it is important to understand the challenges and experiences of breast cancer survivors.

2. What are the key components for promoting quality of life for breast cancer survivors?

3. What are the challenges for providing comprehensive and supportive care for breast cancer survivors?

A FINAL WORD

In 2022, over 20,000 Australians were diagnosed with breast cancer. This chronic disease requires long-term management of side effects from treatment, both physically and psychologically, and the risk of recurrence never goes away completely. In addition to receiving a cancer diagnosis, the cancer treatment and its long-term side effects can also be overwhelming and traumatising experiences. Providing adequate support and care to these women and their families is imperative.

All healthcare professionals play an important role in providing supportive care to breast cancer survivors and their families. Through the story that Linda shared about the challenges she experienced during the cancer journey from the patient's perspective and through Joey's story, whose experience was from a physiotherapist's perspective, we hope you have been given insights into the importance of person-centred care and what services and resources are needed to support breast cancer survivors in order to promote their quality of life.

References and further reading

Chapter 1

Australian Institute of Health and Welfare (AIHW). (2020). Australia's health 2020. Cat. No. AUS 232. AIHW.

Australian Institute of Health and Welfare (AIHW). (2021). Chronic conditions and multimorbidity. AIHW. https://www.aihw.gov.au/reports/chronic-disease/chronic-condition-multimorbidity/contents/chronic-conditions-and-multimorbidity

Fifty-Fourth World Health Assembly. (2001). International classification of functioning, disability and health. http://apps.who.int/gb/archive/pdf_files/WHA54/ea54r21.pdf?ua=1

Chang, E., & Johnson, A. (2022). *Living with chronic illness and disability: Principles for nursing practice* (4th ed.). Elsevier.

Larson, P. (2016). Chronicity. In P. D. Larsen (Ed.), *Lubkin's chronic illness: Impact and interventions* (9th ed.). Jones and Bartlett Learning.

Larson, P. (2019). Chronicity. In P. D. Larsen (Ed.), *Lubkin's chronic illness: Impact and interventions* (10th ed.). Jones and Bartlett Learning.

Ministry of Health (MoH). (2012). *Implementing the New Zealand health strategy 2011*. Ministry of Health. https://www.health.govt.nz/about-ministry/corporate-publications/implementing-new-zealand-health-strategy

World Health Organization (WHO). (2008). 2008–2013 Action plan for the global strategy for the prevention and control of noncommunicable diseases. https://www.who.int/publications/i/item/9789241597418

World Health Organization (WHO). (2011). World report on disability. https://www.who.int/teams/noncommunicable-diseases/sensory-functions-disability-and-rehabilitation/world-report-on-disability

World Health Organization (WHO). (2013). Global action plan for the prevention and control of NCDs 2013–2020. https://www.who.int/publications/i/item/9789241506236

World Health Organization (WHO). (2014). Global Status report on noncommunicable diseases. https://apps.who.int/iris/bitstream/handle/10665/148114/9789241564854_eng.pdf

FURTHER READING

Johnson, A., & Chang, E. (2022). Chronic illness and disability: An overview. In E. Chang, & A. Johnson (Eds.), *Living with chronic illness and disability: Principles for nursing practice* (4th ed.). Elsevier.

Mather, C., & Almond, H. C. (2023). Critically reflective practice for the graduate. In E. Chang, & D. Hatcher (Eds.), *Transitions in nursing: Preparing for professional practice* (6th ed.). Elsevier.

Rolley, J. X., Chang, E., & Johnson, A. (2022). Spirituality. In E. Chang, & A. Johnson (Eds.), *Living with chronic illness and disability: Principles for nursing practice* (4th ed.). Elsevier.

Stein-Parbury, J., & Zugai, J. (2023). Communication for effectiveness. In E. Chang, & D. Hatcher (Eds.), *Transitions in nursing: Preparing for professional practice* (6th ed.). Elsevier.

Wilson, N. J., & Charnock, D. (2022). Health disparities and people with intellectual and developmental disability. In E. Chang, & A. Johnson (Eds.), *Living with chronic illness and disability: Principles for nursing practice* (4th ed.). Elsevier.

World Health Organization (WHO). (2020). *Noncommunicable diseases progress monitor 2020*. WHO. https://www.who.int/publications/i/item/9789240000490

WEBSITES

Blue zones: bluezones.com

Top ways to prevent and reduce chronic disease: accesshc.org.au/resources/top-ways-to-prevent-and-reduce-chronic-disease/

Chapter 2

Aschoff, A., Kremer, P., Hashemi, B., & Kunze, S. (1999). The scientific history of hydrocephalus and its treatment. *Neurosurgical Review, 22*, 67–93. https://doi.org/10.1007/s101430050035

Cashin, A., Pracilio, A., Buckley, T., Kersten, M., Trollor, J., Morphet, J., Howie, V., & Wilson, N. J. (2021). A survey of Australian Registered Nurses' educational experiences and self-perceived capability to care for people with intellectual disability and/or autism. *Journal of Intellectual and Developmental Disability, 47*(3), 227–239. https://doi.org/10.3109/13668250.2021.1967897

Christensen, L. L., Fraynt, R. J., Neece, C. L., & Baker, B. L. (2012). Bullying adolescents with intellectual disability. *Journal of Mental Health Research in Intellectual Disabilities, 5*(1), 49–65. https://doi.org/10.1080/19315864.2011.637660

Desroches, M. (2020). Nurses' attitudes, beliefs, and emotions toward caring for adults with intellectual disabilities: An integrative review. *Nursing Forum, 55*(2), 211–222. https://doi.org/10.1111/nuf.12418

Hansji, N., Wilson, N. J., & Cordier, R. (2015). Men's Sheds: Enabling environments for Australian men living with long-term disabilities. *Health and Social Care in the Community, 23*(3), 272–281. https://doi.org/10.1111/hsc.12140

Hong, S., Yang, J., Kim, D., & Lee, Y. (2022). Accessible guide for people with intellectual disabilities in a fitness environment: A Delphi study. *Adapted Physical Activity Quarterly*. https://doi.org/10.1123/apaq.2022-0036

Hunter, K. F., Bharmal, A., & Moore, K. N. (2013). Long-term bladder drainage: Suprapubic catheter versus other methods: A scoping review. *Neurourology and Urodynamics, 32*(7), 944–951. https://doi.org/10.1002/nau.22356

ICF Education. (2022). *What is ICF?* http://icfeducation.org/what-is-icf

Lewis, P., Gaffney, R. J., & Wilson, N. J. (2017). A narrative review of acute care nurses' experiences nursing patients with intellectual disability: Underprepared, communication barriers and ambiguity about the role of caregivers. *Journal of Clinical Nursing, 26*(11–12), 1473–1484. https://doi.org/10.1111/jocn.13512

Wilson, N. J., & Charnock, D. (2022). Health disparities and people with intellectual and developmental disability. In E. Chang, & A. Johnson (Eds.), *Living with chronic illness and disability: Principles for nursing practice* (4th ed, pp. 115–132). Elsevier.

Wilson, N. J., & Cordier, R. (2013). A narrative review of Men's Sheds literature: Reducing social isolation and promoting men's health and wellbeing. *Health and Social Care in the Community, 21*(5), 451–463. https://doi.org/10.1111/hsc.12019

Wilson, N. J., Cordier, R., Parsons, R., Vaz, S., & Buchanan, A. (2016). Men with disabilities: A cross sectional survey of health promotion, social inclusion and participation at community Men's Sheds. *Disability and Health Journal, 9*(1), 118–126. https://doi.org/10.1016/j.dhjo.2015.08.013

Wilson, N. J., Stancliffe, R. J., Gambin, N., Craig, D., Bigby, C., & Balandin, S. (2015). A case study about the supported participation of older men with lifelong disabilities at Australian community-based Men's Sheds. *Journal of Intellectual and Developmental Disability, 40*(4), 330–341. https://doi.org/10.3109/13668250.2015.1051522

World Health Organization (WHO). (2001). *The International Classification of Functioning, Disability and Health (ICF)*. WHO. https://www.who.int/standards/classifications/international-classification-of-functioning-disability-and-health

Xu, T., & Stancliffe, R. J. (2019). An evaluation of employment outcomes achieved by transition to work service providers in Sydney, Australia. *Journal of Intellectual and Developmental Disability, 44*(1), 51–63. https://doi.org/10.3109/13668250.2017.1310809

Chapter 3

Sattler, L., Hing, W., & Vertullo, C. (2020). Changes to rehabilitation after total knee replacement. *Australian Journal of General Practice, 49*(9), 587–591.

Wall, C., & de Steiger, R. (2020). Pre-operative optimisation for hip and knee arthroplasty: Minimise risk and maximise recovery. *Australian Journal of General Practice, 49*(11), 711–714.

Wall, C., Johnson, T., & de Steiger, R. (2020). Symptom management for patients awaiting joint replacement surgery. *Australian Journal of General Practice, 49*(7), 444–446.

FURTHER READING

Agency for Clinical Innovation (ACI). (2017). *Rehabilitation for chronic conditions.* ACI Rehabilitation for Chronic Conditions Working Group. https://aci.health.nsw.gov.au/__data/assets/pdf_file/0006/385998/ACI-Rehabilitation-for-chronic-conditions-framework.pdf

Agency for Healthcare Research and Quality (AHRQ). (2020). *Prehabilitation and rehabilitation for major joint replacement surgery.* US Department of Health & Human Services. https://effectivehealthcare.ahrq.gov/products/major-joint-replacement/protocol

Health, SA (2016). *Clinical services capability framework: Rehabilitation services.* Department for Health and Ageing, Government of South Australia. https://www.sahealth.sa.gov.au/wps/wcm/connect/09a8b3804e49fa3f9249dac09343dd7f/15137.3-26+Rehab+Services-Sec.pdf?MOD=AJPERES&CACHEID=ROOTWORKSPACE-09a8b3804e49fa3f9249dac09343dd7f-nK6hwcJ

Dávila Castrodad, I. M., Recai, T. M., Abraham, M. M., Etcheson, J. I., Mohamed, N. S., Edalatpour, A., & Delanois, R. E. (2019). Rehabilitation protocols following total knee arthroplasty: A review of study designs and outcome measures. *Annals of Translational Medicine, 7*(Suppl 7), S255. https://doi.org/10.21037/atm.2019.08.15

Pryor, J., O'Reilly, K., Bonser, M., Garrett, G., & McKechnie, D. (2022). Principles for nursing practice: Rehabilitation for the individual and family. In E. Chang, & A. Johnson (Eds.), *Living with Chronic Illness and Disability: Principles for nursing practice* (4th ed.). Elsevier.

WEBSITE

Aruna Rehabilitation Service: https://arunarehab.com.au

Chapter 4

Australia Institute of Health and Welfare. (2022). Cancer data in Australia. *Web report.* https://www.aihw.gov.au/reports/cancer/cancer-data-in-australia/contents/survival

Gaze, M. N., & Wilson, I. M. (2003). *Handbook of Community Cancer Care.* Greenwich Medical Media (GMM) Limited.

World Health Organization (WHO). (2022a). *Palliative care.* WHO. https://www.who.int/health-topics/palliative-care

World Health Organization (WHO). (2022b). WHO launches new campaign to amplify the lived experience of people affected by cancer. *Health Topics.* https://www.who.int/news/item/18-10-2022-who-launches-new-campaign-to-amplify-the-lived-experience-of-people-affected-by-cancer

FURTHER READING

Australian College of Nursing. (2019). Achieving Quality Palliative Care for All: The essential role of nurses (a white paper). CAN.

Cancer Australia. (2010–2014). Psychosocial guidelines. Australian Government. https://www.canceraustralia.gov.au/clinicians-hub/psychosocial-care/psychosocial-guidelines

Goldsbury, D. E., Weber, M. F., Yap, S., Rankin, N. M., Ngo, P., Veerman, L., Banks, E., Canfell, K., & O'Connell, D. L. (2020). Health services costs for lung cancer care in Australia: Estimates from the 45 and Up study. *PloS One, 15*(8), e0238018. 10.1371/journal.pone.0238018

Holden, C. E., Wheelwright, S., Harle, A., & Wagland, R. (2021). The role of health literacy in cancer care: A mixed studies systematic review. *PloS One, 16*(11), e0259815. 10.1371/journal.pone.0259815

Vanstone, M., Canfield, C., Evans, C., Leslie, M., Levasseur, M. A., MacNeil, M., Pahwa, M., Panday, J., Rowland, P., Taneja, S., Tripp, L., You, J., & Abelson, J. (2023). Towards conceptualising patients as partners in health systems: a systematic review and descriptive synthesis. *Health Research Policy and Systems, 21*(12). https://doi.org/10.1186/s12961-022-00954-8

Zhou, K., & Fu, J. (2022). Evolution of oncology and palliative nursing in meeting the changing landscape of cancer care. *Journal of Healthcare Engineering, 2022*, 1–8. https://doi.org/10.1155/2022/3831705

WEBSITES

Cancer Australia: https://www.canceraustralia.gov.au/

Cancer Council: https://www.cancer.org.au/

Conquer magazine: https://conquer-magazine.com/

Optimal Care Pathways: https://www.cancer.org.au/health-professionals/optimal-cancer-care-pathways

Specifically, refer to the *Optimal Care Pathway for People with Lung Cancer*, 2nd ed.

Chapter 5

Australian College of Mental Health Nurses (ACMHN). (2018). *Mental health practice standards for nurses in Australian general practice*. ACMHN.

Australian Institute of Health and Welfare (AIHW). (2022). *Specialist homelessness services annual report 2021–22.* https://www.aihw.gov.au/reports/homelessness-services/specialist-homelessness-services-annual-report

Batterbee, R. (2022). Principles for nursing practice: Depression. In E. Chang, & A. Johnson (Eds.), *Living with chronic illness and disability: Principles for nursing practice* (4th ed.). Elsevier.

Brackertz, N., Borrowman, L., Roggenbuck, C., Pollock, S., & Davis, E. (2020). *Trajectories: The interplay between housing and mental health pathways*. Australian Housing and Urban Research Institute Limited. https://www.ahuri.edu.au/housing/trajectories

Burns, V. F., & Sussman, T. (2019). Homeless for the first time in later life: Uncovering more than one pathway. *The Gerontologist, 59*(2), 251–259. https://doi.org/10.1093/geront/gnx212

Canavan, R., Barry, M. M., Matanov, A., Barros, H., Gabor, E., Greacen, T., Holcnerová, Kluge, U., Nicaise, P., Moskalewicz, J., Díaz-Olalla, J. M., Straßmayr, C., Schene, A. H., Soares, J. J. F., Gaddini, A., & Priebe, S (2012). Service provision and barriers to care for homeless people with mental health problems across 14 European capital cities. *BMC Health Services Research, 12*(222). https://doi.org/10.1186/1472-6963-12-222

Chang, O., Patel, V. L., Iyengar, S., & May, W. (2021). Impact of a mobile-based (mHealth) tool to support community health nurses in early identification of depression and suicide risk in Pacific Island Countries. *Australasian Psychiatry, 29*(2), 200–203. https://doi.org/10.1177/1039856220956458

McInnes, S., Halcomb, E., Ashley, C., Kean, A., Moxham, L., & Patterson, C. (2022). An integrative review of primary health care nurses' mental health knowledge gaps and learning needs. *Collegian, 29*(4), 540–548. https://doi.org/10.1016/j.colegn.2021.12.005

Meehan, T., Baker, D., Blyth, D., & Stedman, T. (2021). Repeat presentations to the emergency department for non-fatal suicidal behaviour: Perceptions of patients. *International Journal of Mental Health Nursing, 30*(1), 200–207. https://doi.org/10.1111/inm.12773

Ngune, I., Hasking, P., McGough, S., Wynaden, D., Janerka, C., & Rees, C. (2021). Perceptions of knowledge, attitude and skills about non-suicidal self-injury: A survey of emergency and mental health nurses. *International Journal of Mental Health Nursing, 30*(3), 635–642. https://doi.org/10.1111/inm.12825

Nursing and Midwifery Board of Australia (NMBA). (2016). *Registered nurse standards for practice.* https://www.nursingmidwiferyboard.gov.au/codes-guidelines-statements/professional-standards/registered-nurse-standards-for-practice.aspx

Petersen, M., Parsell, C., Phillips, R., & White, G. (2014). *Preventing first time homelessness amongst older Australians.* AHURI Final Report No. 222, Australian Housing and Urban Research Institute Limited. https://www.ahuri.edu.au/research/final-reports/222

Polacsek, M., Boardman, G. H., & McCann, T. V. (2019). Help-seeking experiences of older adults with a diagnosis of moderate depression. *International Journal of Mental Health Nursing, 28*(1), 278–287. https://doi.org/10.1111/inm.12531

Rawson, H., Bennett, P. N., Ockerby, C., Hutchinson, A. M., & Considine, J. (2017). Emergency nurses' knowledge and self-rated practice skills when caring for older patients in the Emergency Department. *Australasian Emergency Nursing Journal, 20*(4), 174–180. https://doi.org/10.1016/j.aenj.2017.08.001

Thredgold, C., Beer, A., Zufferey, C., Peters, A., & Spinney, A. (2019). *An effective homelessness services system for older Australians, AHURI Final Report No. 322.* Australian Housing and Urban Research Institute Limited. doi:10.18408/ahuri-7318601. https://www.ahuri.edu.au/research/final-reports/322

FURTHER READING

Dawel, A., Shou, Y., Smithson, M., Cherbuin, N., Banfield, M., Calear, A. L., Farrer, L. M., Gray, D., Gulliver, A., Housen, T., McCallum, S. M., Morse, A. R., Murray, K., Newman, E., Rodney Harris, R. M., & Batterham, P. J. (2020). The effect of COVID-19 on mental health and wellbeing in a representative sample of Australian adults. *Frontiers in Psychiatry, 11.* https://doi.org/10.3389/fpsyt.2020.579985

Eidam, C. (2020). Depression and nursing. *American Journal of Nursing, 120*(10), 13. https://doi.org/10.1097/01.NAJ.0000718544.02650.d9

Flatau, P., Conroy, E., Thielking, M., Clear, A., Hall, S., Bauskis, A., & Farrugia, M. (2013). *How integrated are homelessness, mental health and drug and alcohol services in Australia? AHURI Final Report No. 206.* Australian Housing and Urban Research Institute Limited. https://doi.org/10.18408/ahuri-8201301. https://www.ahuri.edu.au/research/final-reports/206

Foulds, J. A., & Lubman, D. I. (2017). Treating depression in patients with alcohol or drug use disorders: A need for clearer guidelines. *Australian & New Zealand Journal of Psychiatry, 51*(7), 668–669. https://doi.org/10.1177/0004867417708611

Grundberg, Å., Hansson, A., Hillerås, P., & Religa, D. (2016). District nurses' perspectives on detecting mental health problems and promoting mental health among community-dwelling seniors with multimorbidity. *Journal of Clinical Nursing, 25*(17–18), 2590–2599. https://doi.org/10.1111/jocn.13302

Hoffman, A., Camac, A., Brown, M. A., Zekry, A., Gellatley, W., Dowdell, L., Francois, R., & Boston, B. (2019). Medical complications of homelessness: A neglected side of men's health. *Internal Medicine Journal, 49*(4), 455–460. https://doi.org/10.1111/imj.14139

Kerrison, S. A., & Chapman, R. (2007). What general emergency nurses want to know about mental health patients presenting to their emergency department. *Accident and Emergency Nursing, 15*(1), 48–55.

Onapa, H., Sharpley, C. F., Bitsika, V., McMillan, M. E., MacLure, K., Smith, L., & Agnew, L. L. (2022). The physical and mental health effects of housing homeless people: A systematic review. *Health & Social Care in the Community, 30*(2), 448–468. https://doi.org/10.1111/hsc.13486

Roy, D. E., & Giddings, L. S. (2022). Principles for nursing practice: Stigmatisation of people living with a chronic illness or disability. In E. Chang, & A. Johnson (Eds.), *Living with chronic illness and disability: Principles for nursing practice* (4th ed.). Elsevier.

WEBSITES

The Australian College of Mental Health Nurses. Publishes guidance and standards for all nurses working with people with mental health issues: https://acmhn.org/Web/Web/Resources/Best-practice-resources.aspx?hkey=c59b34ff-f05a-46a1-9b27-accc4288813b

Australian Housing and Urban Research Institute Limited. Delivers and disseminates research around housing, homelessness, cities and related urban outcomes: https://www.ahuri.edu.au/

Australian Institute of Health and Welfare. Reports on the statistics relating to the health and social care of homeless people in Australia: https://www.aihw.gov.au/reports/homelessness-services/specialist-homelessness-services-annual-report

Beyond Blue. Provides online resources for depression and other mental illness: https://www.beyondblue.org.au/the-facts/depression?gclid=EAIaIQobChMIzN7RqvmI-AIVizgrCh0m_QPtEAAYASAAEgINKPD_BwE

Head to Health. An online suite of mental health resources for individuals and professionals: https://www.headtohealth.gov.au/search-resources

Chapter 6

Kitwood, T. (1990). The dialectics of dementia: With particular reference to Alzheimer's Disease. *Ageing and Society, 10*(2), 177–196. 10.1017/s0144686×00008060

Kitwood, T. (1997). *Dementia reconsidered: The person comes first.* Open University Press.

Kitwood, T., & Bredin, K. (1992). Towards a theory of dementia care: Personhood and well-being. *Ageing and Society, 12*, 269–287. https://doi.org/10.1017/S0144686×0000502X

Lee, K., Chung, J., Meyer, K. N., & Dionne-Odom, J. N. (2022). Unmet needs and health-related quality of life of dementia family caregivers transitioning from home to long-term care: A scoping review. *Geriatric Nursing, 43*, 254–264. https://doi.org/10.1016/j.gerinurse.2021.12.005

Nolan, M., Brown, J., Davies, S., Nolan, J., & Keady, J. (2006). *The senses framework: Improving care for older people through a relationship-centred approach* (1-902411-44-7). https://shura.shu.ac.uk/280/1/PDF%20Senses%20Framework_Report.pdf

Nolan, M., Davies, S., Brown, J., Keady, J., & Nolan, J. (2004). Beyond 'person-centred' care: A new vision for gerontological nursing. *Journal of Clinical Nursing, 13*(s1), 45–53. https://doi.org/10.1111/j.1365-2702.2004.00926.x

Royal Commission into Aged Care Quality and Safety. (2021). *Final report: Care, dignity and respect.* Commonwealth of Australia. https://agedcare.royalcommission.gov.au/sites/default/files/2021-03/final-report-volume-1_0.pdf

FURTHER READING

Chang, E., & Johnson, A. (2022). Principles for nursing practice: Advanced dementia. In E. Chang, & A, Johnson (Eds.), *Living with chronic illness and disability: Principles for nursing practice* (4th ed.). Elsevier.

Hennelly, N., & O'Shea, E. (2022). A multiple perspective view of personhood in dementia. *Ageing and Society, 42*, 2103–2121. https://doi.org/10.1017/S0144686×20002007

WEBSITE

You may now like to take the opportunity to review some of the additional subject guides and library resources, including fiction and non-fiction books, available at Dementia Australia: dementia-org.libguides.com/home

Chapter 7

ABS (Australian Bureau of Statistics). (2019a). *Disability, ageing and carers, Australia: Summary of findings, 2018.* Australian Government. https://www.abs.gov.au/statistics/health/disability/disability-ageing-and-carers-australia-summary-findings/latest-release

Australian Bureau of Statistics (ABS). (2019b). *Household and family projections, Australia, 2016–2041.* ABS. https://www.abs.gov.au/statistics/people/population/household-and-family-projections-australia/latest-release

Australian Institute of Health and Welfare (AIHW). (2017). *Australia's welfare 2017: In brief.* Australian Government. https://www.aihw.gov.au/reports/australias-welfare/australias-welfare-2017-in-brief/contents/about

Australian Institute of Health and Welfare (AIHW). (2021). *Informal carers*. Australian Government. https://www.aihw.gov.au/reports/australias-welfare/informal-carers

Carers Australia. (2022). Caring costs us: The economic impact on lifetime income and retirement savings of informal carers. https://www.carersaustralia.com.au/caring-costs-us/

Deloitte Access Economics. (2020). The value of informal care in 2020. Carers Australia. https://www.carersaustralia.com.au/wp-content/uploads/2020/07/FINAL-Value-of-Informal-Care-22-May-2020_No-CIC.pdf

Denham, A. M. J., Wynne, O., Baker, A. L., Spratt, N. J., Loh, M., Turner, A., Magin, P., & Bonevski, B. (2022). The long-term unmet needs of informal carers of stroke survivors at home: A systematic review of qualitative and quantitative studies. *Disability and Rehabilitation, 44*(1), 1–12. https://doi.org/10.1080/09638288.2020.1756470

Gérain, P., & Zech, E. (2019). Informal caregiver burnout? Development of a theoretical framework to understand the impact of caregiving. *Frontiers in Psychology, 10*, 1748. https://doi.org/10.3389/fpsyg.2019.01748

House of Representatives Standing Committee on Family, Community, Housing and Youth. (2009). *'Who Cares…?: Report on inquiry into better support for carers*. Commonwealth of Australia. https://www.aph.gov.au/parliamentary_business/committees/house_of_representatives_committees?url=fchy/carers/report.htm

Triantafillou, J., Naiditch, M., Repkova, K., Stiehr, K., Carretero, S., Emilsson, T., Di Santo, P., Bednarik, L., Ceruzzi, F., Cordero, L., Mastroyiannakis, T., Ferrando, M., Mingot, K., Ritter, J., & Viantoni, D. (2010). Informal care in the long-term care system: European Overview Paper. *European Centre for Social Welfare Policy and Research*. https://www.euro.centre.org/downloads/detail/768

Zhu, L., Heffernan, C., & Jie, T. (2020). Caregiver burden: A concept analysis. *International Journal of Nursing Sciences, 7*(4). https://doi.org/10.1016/j.ijnss.2020.07.012

FURTHER READING

Department of Health. (2019). *Home care packages program data report, 1st Quarter 2019–20*. https://www.gen-agedcaredata.gov.au/Resources/Reports-and-publications/2019/December/Home-care-packages-program-data-report-1-July-%E2%80%93-30

Ferguson, C. (2022). Principles for nursing practice: Stroke. In E. Chang, & A. Johnson (Eds.), *Living with chronic illness and disability: Principles for nursing practice* (4th ed.). Elsevier.

Lutz, B. J., Young, M. E., Cox, K. J., Martz, C., & Creasy, K. R. (2011). The crisis of stroke: Experiences of patients and their family caregivers. *Topics in Stroke Rehabilitation, 18*(6), 786–797. https://doi.org/10.1310/tsr1806-786

Productivity Commission. (2011). *Caring for older Australians*. Australian Government.

Productivity Commission. (2020). *Report on government services 2020*. https://www.pc.gov.au/ongoing/report-on-government-services/2020

Stina, L., Carstensen, K., Jørgensen, C. R., & Nielsen, C. P. (2017). Stroke patients' and informal carers' experiences with life after stroke: An overview of qualitative systematic reviews. *Disability and Rehabilitation, 39*(3), 301–313. https://doi.org/10.3109/09638288.2016.1140836

WEBSITES

Carers Australia: www.carersaustralia.com.au

Stroke Foundation Australia: https://strokefoundation.org.au/– 'Inform me' is the platform for health professionals on the Stroke Foundation website and 'Enable me' is the platform for stroke survivors and carers.

Chapter 8

Alkhaqani, A. L. (2022). Importance of teamwork communication in nursing practice. *Nursing Communications, 6*(e2022015), 1–2.

Allen, C. (2022). Principles for nursing practice: Persistent asthma. In Chang, E. & Johnson, A. (Eds.), *Living with chronic illness and disability: Principles for nursing practice* (4th ed.). Elsevier.

Chichirez, C. M., & Purcărea, V. L. (2018). Interpersonal communication in healthcare. *Journal of Medicine and Life, 11*(2), 119–122.

Easey, D., Reddel, H. K., Foster, J. M., Kirkpatrick, S., Locock, L., Ryan, K., & Smith, L. (2019). '… I've said I wish I was dead, you'd be better off without me': A systematic review of people's experiences of living with severe asthma. *Journal of Asthma, 56*(3), 311–322.

Garner, O., Ramey, J. S., & Hanania, N. A. (2022). Management of life-threatening asthma: Severe asthma series. *Chest, 162*(4), 747–756. https://doi.org/10.1016/j.chest.2022.02.029

George, M., Graff, C., Bombezin–Domino, A., & Pain, E (2022). Patients with severe uncontrolled asthma: Perception of asthma control and its management. *Pulmonary Therapy, 8*(2), 209–223.

Global Initiative for Asthma (GINA). (2022). *2022 GINA Report, Global strategy for asthma management and prevention.* https://ginasthma.org/gina-reports/

Hiles, S. A., Urroz, P. D., Gibson, P. G., Bogdanovs, A., & McDonald, V. M. (2021). A feasibility randomised controlled trial of Novel Activity Management in severe ASthma-Tailored Exercise (NAMASTE): Yoga and mindfulness. *BMC Pulmonary Medicine, 21*(71). https://doi.org/10.1186/s12890-021-01436-3

Holst, S. S., Sabedin, E., Sabedin, E., & Vermehren, C. (2023). A shift in asthma treatment according to new guidelines: An evaluation of asthma patients' attitudes towards treatment change. *International Journal of Environmental Research and Public Health, 20*(4), 3453. https://doi.org/10.3390/ijerph20043453

Majellano, E. C., Clark, V. L., Foster, J. M., Gibson, P. G., & McDonald, V. M. (2021). 'It's like being on a roller coaster': the burden of caring for people with severe asthma. *ERJ Open Research, 7*(2).

Majellano, E. C., Clark, V. L., McLoughlin, R. F., Gibson, P. G., & McDonald, V. M. (2022). Using a knowledge translation framework to identify health care professionals' perceived barriers and enablers for personalised severe asthma care. *PloS one, 17*(6), e0269038.

McDonald, V. M., Clark, V. L., & Gibson, P. G. (2022). 'Nothing about us without us'—What matters to patients with severe asthma? *The Journal of Allergy and Clinical Immunology: In Practice, 10*(3), 890–891.

McDonald, V. M., Hiles, S. A., Jones, K. A., Clark, V. L., & Yorke, J. (2018). Health-related quality of life burden in severe asthma. *Medical Journal of Australia, 209*(S2), S28–S33.

Nanda, A., & Wasan, A. N. (2020). Asthma in adults. *Medical Clinics, 104*(1), 95–108.

Papi, A., Blasi, F., Canonica, G. W., Morandi, L., Richeldi, L., & Rossi, A. (2020). Treatment strategies for asthma: Reshaping the concept of asthma management. *Allergy, Asthma & Clinical Immunology, 16*(75). https://doi.org/10.1186/s13223-020-00472-8

Salazar, L. R. (2018). The effect of patient self-advocacy on patient satisfaction: Exploring self-compassion as a mediator. *Communication Studies, 69*(5), 567–582. https://doi.org/10.1080/10510974.2018.1462224

Schena, D., Rosales, R., & Rowe, E. (2022). Teaching self-advocacy skills: A review and call for research. *Journal of Behavioral Education.* https://doi.org/10.1007/s10864-022-09472-7

Schuckmann, K. (2022). *Factors affecting quality of life and asthma control in older adults with asthma.* Electronic Theses and Dissertations. Paper 3807. https://doi.org/10.18297/etd/3807

Stubbs, M. A., Clark, V. L., Cheung, M., Smith, L., Saini, B., Yorke, J., Majellano, E. C., Gibson, P. G., & McDonald, V. M. (2021). The experience of living with severe asthma, depression and anxiety: A qualitative art-based study. *Journal of Asthma and Allergy, 14*, 1527–1537. https://doi.org/10.2147/JAA.S328104

Stubbs, M. A., Clark, V. L., & McDonald, V. M. (2019). Living well with severe asthma. *Breathe (Sheff), 15*(2), e40–e49. https://doi.org/10.1183/20734735.0165-2019

Walker, S. (2022). Patient advocacy: An antidote to loneliness and more. *BMJ Medicine, 1*(1), e000194. https://doi.org/10.1136/bmjmed-2022-000194

FURTHER READING

Clark, V. L., Gibson, P. G., Genn, G., Hiles, S. A., Pavord, I. D., & McDonald, V. M. (2017). Multidimensional assessment of severe asthma: A systematic review and meta-analysis. *Respirology (Carlton, Vic.), 22*(7), 1262–1275. https://doi.org/10.1111/resp.13134

Holguin, F., Cardet, J. C., Chung, K. F., Diver, S., Ferreira, D. S., Fitzpatrick, A., Gaga, M., Kellermeyer, L., Khurana, S., Knight, S., McDonald, V. M., Morgan, R. L., Ortega, V. E., Rigau, D., Subbarao, P., Tonia, T., Adcock, I. M., Bleecker, E. R., Brightling, C., … Bush, A. (2020). Management of severe asthma: A European Respiratory Society/American Thoracic Society guideline. *European Respiratory Journal, 55*(1). https://doi.org/10.1183/13993003.00588-2019

WEBSITES

American Thoracic Society (ATS): https://www.thoracic.org

Asthma and Allergy Foundation of America: https://www.aafa.org

Asthma and Lung UK: https://www.asthma.org.uk

Asthma Australia: https://asthma.org.au

Asthma First Aid: https://asthma.org.au/treatment-diagnosis/asthma-first-aid/

Asthma New Zealand: https://www.asthma.org.nz

Asthma WA: https://asthmawa.org.au

Australian College of Nursing: https://www.acn.edu.au

Covid Healthcare Survey 2021: https://asthma.org.au/wp-content/uploads/2021/08/Access-to-healthcare-summary_Media-.pdf

Global Initiative for Asthma (GINA): https://ginasthma.org

Healthtalk Australia: https://www.healthtalkaustralia.org

The National Asthma Council Australia: https://www.nationalasthma.org.au

Severe Asthma Toolkit: https://toolkit.severeasthma.org.au

Severe Asthma Toolkit Overview: https://youtu.be/fUFAL4szQQQ

Treatable Traits: https://treatabletraits.org.au

Chapter 9

Akhmedov, A., & Narziev, L. (2023). Predictors of cardiovascular complications in patients with chronic ischemic heart disease after bypass surgery. *International Journal of Medical Sciences and Clinical Research, 3*(3), 68–77.

Akpinar, F. M., & Oral, A. (2023). Does exercise-based cardiac rehabilitation reduce mortality and hospitalization rates after heart valve surgery? A Cochrane Review summary with commentary. *American Journal of Physical Medicine & Rehabilitation, 102*(2), 169–171.

Al-Omary, M. (2021). *Heart failure outcomes in Hunter New England area between 2005–2014.* University of Newcastle.

Aluru, J. S., Barsouk, A., Saginala, K., Rawla, P., & Barsouk, A. (2022). Valvular Heart Disease Epidemiology. *Medical Sciences, 10*(2), 32.

Australian Bureau of Statistics (ABS). (2018). *Disability, ageing and carers, Australia: Summary of findings.* https://www.abs.gov.au/statistics/health/disability/disability-ageing-and-carers-australia-summary-findings/latest-release

Australian Bureau of Statistics (ABS). (2022). *Health conditions prevalence.* ABS. https://www.abs.gov.au/statistics/health/health-conditions-and-risks/health-conditions-prevalence/latest-release

Australian Institute of Health and Welfare (AIHW). (2019). *Cardiovascular disease in women.* https://www.aihw.gov.au/reports/heart-stroke-vascular-diseases/cardiovascular-disease-in-women-main/summary

Beatty, A. L., Beckie, T. M., Dodson, J., Goldstein, C. M., Hughes, J. W., Kraus, W. E., Martin, S. S., Olson, T. P., Pack, Q. R., Stolp, H., Thomas, R. J., Wu, W-C., & Franklin, B. A. (2023). A new era in cardiac rehabilitation delivery: Research gaps, questions, strategies, and priorities. *Circulation, 147*(3), 254–266.

Curtis, E., Fernandez, R., Moroney, T., & Lee, A. (2020). How coronary artery catheterisation has influenced cardiovascular nursing – An historical Australian perspective. *Collegian, 27*(6), 649–653.

Desai, D. S., & Hajouli, S. (2022). *Arrhythmias*. In *StatPearls [Internet]*. StatPearls Publishing.

Dibben, G. O., Faulkner, J., Oldridge, N., Rees, K., Thompson, D. R., Zwisler, A.-D., & Taylor, R. S. (2023). Exercise-based cardiac rehabilitation for coronary heart disease: A meta-analysis. *European Heart Journal, 44*(6), 452–469.

Fernandez, R., Ellwood, L., Lord, H., Curtis, E., Khoo, J., Lee, A., & Weaver, J. (2021). Preprocedural anxiety in the transradial cardiac catheterization era. *Journal of Cardiovascular Nursing, 36*(4), E20–E28.

Gaudino, M., Chadow, D., Rahouma, M., Sandner, S., Perezgrovas-Olaria, R., Audisio, K., Cancelli, G., Bratton, B. A., Fremes, S., Kurlansky, P., Girardi, L., & Habib, R. H. (2023). Operative outcomes of women undergoing coronary artery bypass surgery in the US, 2011 to 2020. *JAMA Surgery, 158*(5), 494–502.

Haider, A., Bengs, S., Luu, J., Osto, E., Siller-Matula, J. M., Muka, T., & Gebhard, C. (2020). Sex and gender in cardiovascular medicine: Presentation and outcomes of acute coronary syndrome. *European Heart Journal, 41*(13), 1328–1336.

Huang, J., Kumar, S., Toleva, O., & Mehta, P. K. (2022). Mechanisms of coronary ischemia in women. *Current Cardiology Reports, 24*(10), 1273–1285.

Khoja, A., Andraweera, P. H., Lassi, Z. S., Ali, A., Zheng, M., Pathirana, M. M., Aldridge, E., Wittwer, M. R., Chaudhuri, D. D., & Tavella, R. (2023). Risk factors for premature coronary heart disease in women compared to men: Systematic review and meta-analysis. *Journal of Women's Health*. https://doi.org/10.1089/jwh.2022.0517

Laflamme, S. Z., Bouchard, K., Sztajerowska, K., Lalande, K., Greenman, P. S., & Tulloch, H. (2022). Attachment insecurities, caregiver burden, and psychological distress among partners of patients with heart disease. *Plos One, 17*(9), e0269366.

Lambrias, A., Ervin, J., Taouk, Y., & King, T. A. (2023). A systematic review comparing cardiovascular disease among informal carers and non-carers. *International Journal of Cardiology Cardiovascular Risk and Prevention, 16*. https://doi.org/10.1016/j.ijcrp.2023.200174

Mcharo, T. L., Iseselo, M. K., Kahema, S. E., & Tarimo, E. (2023). Experiences of family caregivers in caring for patients with heart failure at Jakaya Kikwete Cardiac Institute, Dar es Salaam, Tanzania: A qualitative study. *medRxiv*. https://doi.org/10.1101/2023.01.12.23284350

Montoy, J. C. C., Shen, Y.-C., & Hsia, R. Y. (2022). Trends in inequities in the treatment of and outcomes for women and minorities with myocardial infarction. *Annals of Emergency Medicine, 80*(2), 108–117.

Sawan, M. A., Calhoun, A. E., Fatade, Y. A., & Wenger, N. K. (2022). Cardiac rehabilitation in women, challenges and opportunities. *Progress in Cardiovascular Diseases, 70*, 111–118.

Sawano, M., Lu, Y., Caraballo, C., Mahajan, S., Dreyer, R., Lichtman, J. H., D'Onofrio, G., Spatz, E., Khera, R., Onuma, O., Murugiah, K., Spertus, J. A., & Krumholz, H. M. (2023). Sex difference in outcomes of acute myocardial infarction in young patients. *Journal of the American College of Cardiology, 81*(18), 1797–1806.

Smith, J. R., Thomas, R. J., Bonikowske, A. R., Hammer, S. M., & Olson, T. P. (2022). Sex differences in cardiac rehabilitation outcomes. *Circulation Research, 130*(4), 552–565.

Stefanakis, M., Batalik, L., Antoniou, V., & Pepera, G. (2022). Safety of home-based cardiac rehabilitation: A systematic review. *Heart & Lung, 55*, 117–126.

Weininger, D., Cordova, J. P., Wilson, E., Eslava, D. J., Alviar, C. L., Korniyenko, A., Bavishi, C. P., Hong, M. K., Chorzempa, A., Fox, J., & Tamis-Holland, J. E. (2022). Delays to hospital presentation in women and men with ST-segment elevation myocardial infarction: A multi-center analysis of patients hospitalized in New York City. *Therapeutics and Clinical Risk Management, 18*, 1–9.

Zhang, W.-Y., Nan, N., He, Y., Zuo, H.-J., Song, X.-T., Zhang, M., & Zhou, Y. (2023). Prevalence of depression and anxiety symptoms and their associations with cardiovascular risk factors in coronary patients. *Psychology, Health & Medicine, 28*(5), 1275–1287.

FURTHER READING

Australian Bureau of Statistics (ABS). (2022). *Causes of death, Australia*, 2021. https://www.abs.gov.au/statistics/health/causes-death/causes-death-australia/latest-release

Australian Bureau of Statistics (ABS). (2022). *Health conditions prevalence*, 2020–21. https://www.abs.gov.au/statistics/health/health-conditions-and-risks/health-conditions-prevalence/latest-release

Australian Institute of Health and Welfare (AIHW). (2023). *Heart, stroke and vascular disease: Australian facts.* AIHW. https://www.aihw.gov.au/reports/heart-stroke-vascular-diseases/hsvd-facts/contents/about

WEBSITES

The Cardiac Society of Australia and New Zealand is the professional body for cardiologists and those working in the area of cardiology, including researchers, scientists, cardiovascular nurses, allied health professionals and other healthcare workers. The Society is the chief advocacy group for the profession and aims to facilitate training, professional development and improve medical practice to enhance the quality of care for patients with cardiovascular disease: https://www.csanz.edu.au/

Carers Australia is the national peak body representing Australia's unpaid carers, advocating on their behalf to influence policies and services at a national level: https://www.carersaustralia.com.au/

Chapter 10

Bonner, A., & Brown, L. (2022). Chronic kidney disease. In E. Chang, & A. Johnson (Eds.), *Living with chronic illness and disability: Principles for nursing practice* (4th ed.). Elsevier.

Bonner, A., Douglas, B., Brown, L., Harvie, B., Lucas, A., Tomlins, M., & Gillespie, K. (2022). Understanding the practice patterns of nephrology nurse practitioners in Australia. *Journal of Renal Care*, 1–10. https://doi.org/10.1111/jorc.12444

Callahan, M. B. (2011). The role of the nephrology social worker in optimizing treatment outcomes for end-stage renal disease patients. *Dialysis & Transplantation, 40*(10), 444–450. https://doi.org/10.1002/dat.20618

de Zeeuw, D. (2008). Renal disease: A common and a silent killer. *Nature Clinical Practice Cardiovascular Medicine, 5*(Suppl 1), S27–S35. https://doi.org/10.1038/ncpcardio0853

Elwyn, G., Coulter, A., Laitner, S., Walker, E., Watson, P., & Thomson, R. (2010). Implementing shared decision making in the NHS. *BMJ, 341*, c5146. https://doi.org/10.1136/bmj.c5146

Fletcher, B. R., Damery, S., Aiyegbusi, O. L., Anderson, N., Calvert, M., Cockwell, P., Ferguson, J., Horton, M., Paap, M. C. S., Sidey-Gibbons, C., Slade, A., Turner, N., & Kyte, D. (2022). Symptom burden and health-related quality of life in chronic kidney disease: A global systematic review and meta-analysis. *PLoS Medicine, 19*, e1003954.

Fu, E. L., Evans, M., Carrero, J., Putter, H., Clase, C. M., Caskey, F. J., Szymczac, M., Torino, C., Chesnaye, N. C., Jager, K. J., Wanner, C., Dekker, F. W., & van Diepen, M. (2021). Timing of dialysis initiation to reduce mortality and cardiovascular events in advanced chronic kidney disease: Nationwide cohort study. *BMJ, 375*, e066306. https://doi.org/10.1136/bmj-2021-066306

Kidney Health Australia. (2023). Your kidneys, retrieved March 29, 2023, from https://kidney.org.au/your-kidneys

Nielsen, C., Clemensen, J., Bistrup, C., & Agerskov, H. Balancing everyday life – Patients' experiences before, during and four months after kidney transplantation. *Nursing Open, 6*(2), 443–452. https://doi.org/10.1002/nop2.225

Nursing and Midwifery Board Australia (NMBA). (2021). *Nurse practitioner standards for practice.* https://www.nursingmidwiferyboard.gov.au/Codes-Guidelines-Statements/Professional-standards/nurse-practitioner-standards-of-practice.aspx

Sargent, J. A., & Gotch, F. A. (1996). Principles and biophysics of dialysis. In C. Jacobs, C. M. Kjellstrand, K. M. Koch, & J. F. Winchester (Eds.), *Replacement of renal function by dialysis.* Springer https://doi.org/10.1007/978-0-585-36947-1_2

Sepúlveda, C., Marlin, A., Yoshida, T., & Ullrich, A. (2002). Palliative care: The World Health Organization's global perspective. *Journal of Pain and Symptom Management, 24*(2), 91–96.

Stevenson, J., Tong, A., Gutman, T., Campbell, K. L., Craig, J. C., Brown, M. A., & Lee, V. W. (2018). Experiences and perspectives of dietary management among patients on hemodialysis: An interview study. *Journal of Renal Nutrition, 28*(6), 411–421. https://doi.org/10.1053/j.jrn.2018.02.005

Transplant Australia. (2023). *FAQ.* https://transplant.org.au/faq/

Tucker, E. L., Smith, A. R., Daskin, M. S., Schapiro, H., Cottrell, S. M., Gendron, E. S., Hill-Callahan, P., Leichtman, A. B., Merion, R. M., Gill, S. J., & Maass, K. L. (2019). Life and expectations post-kidney transplant: A qualitative analysis of patient responses. *BMC Nephrology, 20*(175). https://doi.org/10.1186/s12882-019-1368-0

Verberne, W. R., Stiggelbout, A. M., Bos, W. J. W., & van Delden, J. J. M. (2022). Asking the right questions: towards a person-centered conception of shared decision-making regarding treatment of advanced chronic kidney disease in older patients. *BMC Medical Ethics, 23*(47). https://doi.org/10.1186/s12910-022-00784-x

Wasse, M., & Beathard, G. A. (2019). *Chronic kidney disease, dialysis, and transplantation* (4th ed.). Elsevier.

Webster, A. C., Nagler, E. V., Morton, R. L., & Masson, P. (2017). Chronic kidney disease. *The Lancet, 389*(10075), 1238–1252. https://doi.org/10.1016/S0140-6736(16)32064-5

Woo, B. F. Y., Lee, J. X. Y., & Tam, W. W. S. (2017). The impact of the advanced practice nursing role on quality of care, clinical outcomes, patient satisfaction, and cost in the emergency and critical care settings: a systematic review. *Human Resources for Health, 15*(63). https://doi.org/10.1186/s12960-017-0237-9

Woodside, K. J., Repeck, K. J., Mukhopadhyay, P., Schaubel, D. E., Shahinian, V. B., Saran, R., & Pisoni, R. L. (2021). Arteriovenous vascular access-related procedural burden among incident hemodialysis patients in the United States. *American Journal of Kidney Disorders, 78*(3), 369–379. https://doi.org/10.1053/j.ajkd.2021.01.019

You, Q., Bai, D. X., Wu, C. X., Chen, H., Hou, C. M., & Gao, J. (2022). Prevalence and risk factors of postdialysis fatigue in patients under maintenance hemodialysis: A systematic review and meta-analysis. *Asian Nursing Research, 16*(5), 292–298. https://doi.org/10.1016/j.anr.2022.11.002

Yu, Y.-J., Wu, I.-W., Huang, C.-Y., Hsu, K.-H., Lee, C.-C., Sun, C.-Y., Hsu, H.-J., & Wu, M.-S. (2014). Multidisciplinary predialysis education reduced the inpatient and total medical costs of the first 6 months of dialysis in incident hemodialysis patients. *PLoS ONE, 9*(11), e112820. https://doi.org/10.1371/journal.pone.0112820

Chapter 11

Adu, M. D., Malabu, U. H., Malau-Aduli, A. E., & Malau-Aduli, B. S. (2019). Enablers and barriers to effective diabetes self-management: A multi-national investigation. *PloS One, 14*(6), e0217771.

Alsaleh, F. M., Smith, F. J., Keady, S., & Taylor, K. M. (2010). Insulin pumps: From inception to the present and toward the future. *Journal of Clinical Pharmacy and Therapeutics, 35*(2), 127–138.

Australian Commission on Safety and Quality in Health Care. (2021). *National safety and quality health service standards* (2nd ed.). https://www.safetyandquality.gov.au/sites/default/files/2021-05/national_safety_and_quality_health_service_nsqhs_standards_second_edition_-_updated_may_2021.pdf

Australian Institute of Health and Welfare (AIHW). (2023). *Diabetes: Australian facts.* AIHW. https://www.aihw.gov.au/reports/diabetes/diabetes/contents/about

Craig, L., Sims, R., Glasziou, P., & Thomas, R. (2020). Women's experiences of a diagnosis of gestational diabetes mellitus: A systematic review. *BMC Pregnancy and Childbirth, 20*(1), 1–15.

Davy, C., Bleasel, J., Liu, H., Tchan, M., Ponniah, S., & Brown, A. (2015). Effectiveness of chronic care models: Opportunities for improving healthcare practice and health outcomes: A systematic review. *BMC Health Services Research, 15*(194). https://doi.org/10.1186/s12913-015-0854-8

Department of Health and Aged Care. (2021). *Australian diabetes strategy 2021–2030.* https://www.health.gov.au/resources/publications/australian-national-diabetes-strategy-2021-2030

Department of Health and Aged Care. (2020). *National Strategic framework for chronic conditions.*https://www.health.gov.au/resources/publications/national-strategic-framework-for-chronic-conditions?language=en#:~:text=The%20National%20Strategic%20Framework%20for,and%20management%20of%20chronic%20conditions

Liu, N. F., Brown, A. S., Folias, A. E., Younge, M. F., Guzman, S. J., Close, K. L., & Wood, R. (2017). Stigma in people with type 1 or type 2 diabetes. *Clinical Diabetes, 35*(1), 27–34.

National Diabetes Services Scheme (NDSS). (2020). *National diabetes nurse education framework 2020–2022.* https://www.ndss.com.au/about-diabetes/resources/find-a-resource/national-diabetes-nursing-education-framework/

Nimri, R., Nir, J., & Phillip, M. (2020). Insulin pump therapy. *American Journal of Therapeutics, 27*(1), e30–e41. https://doi.org/10.1097/MJT.0000000000001097

Speight, J., Holmes-Truscott, E., Hendrieckx, C., Skovlund, S., & Cooke, D. J. D. M. (2020). Assessing the impact of diabetes on quality of life: What have the past 25 years taught us? *Diabetic Medicine, 37*(3), 483–492.

FURTHER READING

Diabetes Australia. (2020). *Gestational diabetes in Australia position statement.* https://www.diabetesaustralia.com.au/wp-content/uploads/Gestational-Diabetes-in-Australia-Position-Statement-2020.pdf

McIntyre, H. D., Catalano, P., Zhang, C., Desoye, G., Mathiesen, E. R., & Damm, P. (2019). Gestational diabetes mellitus. *Nature Reviews Disease Primers, 5*(1), 47.

White, H., Tendal, B., Elliott, J., Turner, T., Andrikopoulos, S., & Zoungas, S. (2020). Breathing life into Australian diabetes clinical guidelines. *Medical Journal of Australia, 212*(6), 250–251.

WEBSITES

Diabetes Australia. (2023). Type 1 diabetes: https://www.diabetesaustralia.com.au/about-diabetes/type-1-diabetes/

Diabetes Australia. (2023). Type 2 diabetes: https://www.diabetesaustralia.com.au/about-diabetes/type-2-diabetes/

Diabetes Australia. (2023). Gestational diabetes: https://www.diabetesaustralia.com.au/about-diabetes/gestational-diabetes/

Diabetes Australia. (2023). What is diabetes: https://www.diabetesaustralia.com.au/about-diabetes/what-is-diabetes/

NMBA. (2016). *Registered Nurse standards for practice*: https://www.nursingmidwiferyboard.gov.au/codes-guidelines-statements/professional-standards/registered-nurse-standards-for-practice.aspx

Chapter 12

Cancer Council Australia. (2023a). *Breast cancer.* https://www.cancer.org.au/cancer-information/types-of-cancer/breast-cancer

Cancer Council NSW. (2023b). *Cancer survivorship.* https://www.cancercouncil.com.au/cancer-information/living-well/after-cancer-treatment/adjusting-to-life-after-treatment/who-is-a-cancer-survivor

FURTHER READING

Acebedo, J. C., Haas, B. K., & Hermans, M. (2021). Breast cancer-related lymphedema in Hispanic women: A phenomenological study. *Journal of Transcultural Nursing, 32*(1), 41–49. https://doi.org/10.1177/1043659619891236

Australian Institute of Health and Welfare (AIHW). (2022a). *Cancer.* AIHW. https://www.aihw.gov.au/reports/australias-health/cancer

Australian Institute of Health and Welfare (AIHW). (2022). *Six national health priority areas.* AIHW. https://www.aihw.gov.au/getmedia/78bc02fd-a75e-4f25-a0ae-b27f7bb2a4b2/bdia-c06.pdf.aspx

Breast Cancer Network Australia. (2023). Caring for someone with early breast cancer. https://www.bcna.org.au/understanding-breast-cancer/caring-for-someone-with-early-breast-cancer/

Breast Cancer Now. (2023). How to support someone with breast cancer. https://breastcancernow.org/information-support/facing-breast-cancer/how-support-someone-breast-cancer

Brunet, J., Price, J., & Harris, C. (2022). Body image in women diagnosed with breast cancer: A grounded theory study. *Body Image, 41*, 417–431. https://doi.org/10.1016/j.bodyim.2022.04.012

Cancer Council NSW. (2023). Survivorship care plan. https://www.cancercouncil.com.au/cancer-information/living-well/after-cancer-treatment/follow-up-care/survivorship-care-plans/

Cancer Australia. (2023). *All cancers in Australia*. Cancer Australia. https://www.canceraustralia.gov.au/impacted-cancer/what-cancer/cancer-australia-statistics

Jadidi, A., & Ameri, F. (2022). Social support and meaning of life in women with breast cancer. *Ethiopian Journal of Health Sciences, 32*(4), 709–714. https://doi.org/10.4314/ejhs.v32i4.6

Kwok, C., & White, K. (2011). Cultural and linguistic isolation: The breast cancer experience of Chinese-Australian women – A qualitative study. *Contemporary Nurse, 39*(1), 85–94. https://doi.org/10.5172/conu.2011.39.1.85

Kwok, C., & White, K. (2014). Perceived information needs and social support of Chinese-Australian breast cancer survivors. *Support Care Cancer, 22*(10), 2651–2659. https://doi.org/10.1007/s00520-014-2252-x

Lovelace, D. L., McDaniel, L. R., & Golden, D. (2019). Long-term effects of breast cancer surgery, treatment, and survivor care. *Journal of Midwifery & Women's Health, 64*(6), 713–724. https://doi.org/10.1111/jmwh.13012

McGrath Foundation. (2023). Breast cancer supportive care – Breast cancer support. https://www.mcgrathfoundation.com.au/get-support/find-a-nurse/?gclid=CjwKCAiAr4GgBhBFEiwAgwORreDGx-9g05S8Jxm5JHRl8MoKZlCNw-bDwQZHt4W7mjyru4G2JCmNHxoCNvEQAvD_BwE

Novitarum, L., Siregar, M. F. G., Siregar, F. A., & Lubis, N. L. (2022). Survivor's experience in fighting breast cancer. *Journal of Population Therapeutics and Clinical Pharmacology, 29*(4), e126–e133. https://doi.org/10.47750/jptcp.2022.976

Rajagopal, L., Liamputtong, P., & McBride, K. A. (2019). The lived experience of Australian women living with breast cancer: A meta-synthesis. *Asian Pacific Journal of Cancer Prevention, 20*(11), 3233–3249. https://doi.org/10.31557/APJCP.2019.20.11.3233

Norouzinia, R., Aghabarari, M., Shiri, M., Karimi, M., & Samami, E. (2015). Communication barriers perceived by nurses and patients. *Global Journal of Health Science, 8*(6), 65–74. https://doi.org/10.5539/gjhs.v8n6p65

Survivingbreastcancer.org/ (2023). Breast cancer support – Empower you from day one. https://www.survivingbreastcancer.org/?gclid=CjwKCAiAr4GgBhBFEiwAgwORrTdG2IgoW84uZR7ycW-J1Zud8sI8jq8UPSOaRUXTohlfJ5c9HR7N-hoCpHYQAvD_BwE

World Health Organization (WHO). (2023). Breast cancer. https://www.who.int/news-room/fact-sheets/detail/breast-cancer

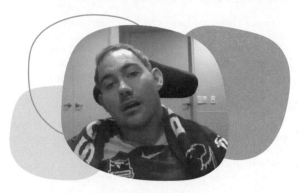

CHAPTER 2

Aaron's story

I have cerebral palsy. Well, I'll start by saying this. I was born with both my hips dislocated. Not long after I was born, I was about three months into my life, I nearly could've died because I was very sick as a result of having 61 different shunt blockages. Let me explain a bit more about that. Because if fluid gets around my brain, it's got the potential to block my shunt. Which could be really fatal. And it could end up in me passing away.

And as I've said, I've already had 61 shunt blockages, but that was all in the first three months of life. And the doctors at that point, they weren't giving me much of a chance to live. But somehow, I survived all of them.

I was originally born in the southwest suburb of Liverpool, Liverpool Hospital. I went to preschool not far down the road from where I was born in Campbelltown, which is Beverley Park in Campbelltown. And then from there, I went to, about 1993, I moved to a school called Broderick in Lakemba at the time. And coming from the southwest, that was a bit of a challenge, because I didn't know what to expect and I felt like I was going to get teased a lot because of what I'd already gone through. But I eventually coped with it. I did get teased quite a bit, but I learned to cope with it and just block it out. Because let's face it, having a disability – being in a wheelchair – is not easy. But it's about making the best out of it that you can. Because at the end of the day, you've only got one life to live. And it's about making the best quality out of it that you possibly can.

A desire for employment

I go to a day program. I'm currently trying to look for a job at the same time. So then it gives me more stability. What I'm saying there is, I want to be able to explore different options as in work. [In the day program] we do everyday life skills, like cooking, going to the gym, sport. We do music. We do a whole bunch of different stuff. At the moment, because I'm into more sport, through them, I've already done a level one coaching course. That was online. And I passed that. Because eventually I want to get a job … I want to try and get into the NRL as a head coach. And I know that's going to be hard, but it's good to have the ambition. I know it's going to have challenges, I understand that. But there's no point setting the goal if you're not going to chase it, you know?

Living with a disability and chronic illness

I'll just say this. [Living with cerebral palsy and hydrocephalus] is a big challenge in my experiences, because not only that but with the dislocated hips and stuff, and not being able to walk, that adds an extra dimension to the challenge that I currently face. Particularly not being able to walk, that's another challenge in itself. In some cases, you'll get some people in the community that say, look at this guy, they'll say, we feel sorry for you. And then I'm like, well, I sort of think how would they like to be in the wheelchair? It's not easy. It's very hard.

Weekly services

In my example, we have OTs – occupational therapists, and also the physiotherapist as well. With the physiotherapist, that's sort of like different exercises. It's like I'm trying to improve the strength that I have. Because at the end of the day, we've got to live all the life as we can. We can't just let the disability get the best of us. That's the wrong way to go about it.

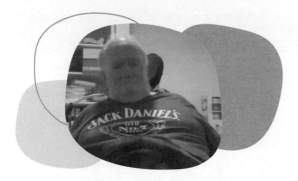

CHAPTER 2

Grant's story

I've got a broken fourth vertebrae. The vertebrae itself is being repaired with two metal plates and eight screws. But after that, now I've got scarring to the spinal cord, which has basically turned me into a quadriplegic. I've got limited movement in my arms and legs.

Health problems

I've got a suprapubic catheter attached to my … it goes straight into my skin to my bladder for my urine. And occasionally there's sediment in the bladder, which blocks up the catheter. And when this happens, I get a UTI (urinary tract infection), and my temperature goes up and I just get an all-around infection. Most times I have to go to the hospital and have an IV antibiotic administered through a cannula for the antibiotic to kill the virus – it usually takes about a week. It can be two or three times a year.

Living with a spinal cord injury

I miss my old lifestyle, not being able to drive a car or socialise properly. That's a bit depressing sometimes, but you have to get over things like that. And learning how to drive a wheelchair and where you can go and can't go. It's all a big learning curve. But in the beginning, I couldn't drive my wheelchair. I had to drive with a chin control because I had limited movement in my arms. But now I can drive with my hands quite all right.

I've always liked things with wheels and motors all my life. I was pretty keen to get mobile and learn how to use it. So it took me about two or three weeks, that's to learn to stop bumping into things and to stay on concrete paths without running off them. But yeah, I'm pretty competent now after five years. I go to shopping centres and back by myself and everything.

Disability-specific social group

[My social life has] gone to practically non-existent now. I'm a member of a disability group that comes and picks me up in a wheelchair bus. You can pick and choose different outings you wish to go on. That's a big benefit to me. Gets me out of the house and I get to go and see different sights and things, that's good.

I haven't got many friends in Sydney, so I've had to make new friends. The boys across the road are my age and similar interests, so I got to know them and we socialise every weekend. That's been a big benefit for me. They're just my neighbours without disabilities.

Therapy to promote wellbeing and independence

Basically, lots of physiotherapy, [has helped with] getting movement back into my limbs again. But when the accident first happened, to transfer from my bed to my wheelchair, I had to use a piece of plastic sheeting and slide from the bed into the wheelchair. But now I've got to the stage where I can stand up and if the carer holds one of my hands, I can walk from my bed to the wheelchair. And I can walk a few steps without anybody holding my hands.

I get up in a walking frame every afternoon and walk up and down the hallway in that, that's a big benefit for me, as far as my leg muscles. And I get weekly visits from my physiotherapist, and that's a big benefit for me as well. And the carers in this accommodation where I am, they've been trained in basic physiotherapy, which they do every afternoon, which is a big benefit. Because with my fingers, they're inclined to cramp up and make a fist, and I can't straighten them out by myself. Because it stays like that, the joints get calcification. New bone growing between the joints. The joints have to be manipulated to break up that new growth and return movement to the joints.

Daily challenges

I don't like getting on public transport. I prefer to catch a wheelchair taxi. Because I don't like the public looking at me getting on and off, I feel a bit intimidated, like everybody's looking at me, embarrassed. So I do it privately in a one-off wheelchair taxi. And I used to feel intimidated going to shopping centres. People staring at me. But now I don't care, it is what it is. And, well, things like not being able to dress myself, not being able to feed myself, not being able to shave, that's all, you know, a big handicap for me, and it's a new lifestyle I have to adapt to.

And especially mosquitoes biting you on the head, you can't brush them away. Lots of different things you have to get used to. You rely on the carers for a lot of help.

A community nurse visits me every Tuesday. And I get my bladder flushed out with Citric Acid Flush. That goes into my bladder for five minutes and then it's drained back out. And at the same time, my blood pressure, temperature, pulse and oxygen levels are all recorded. So I like to know what it is myself.

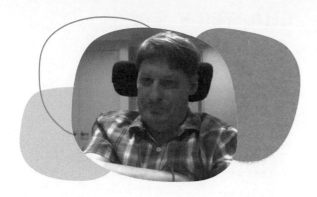

CHAPTER 2

Jamie's story

My name is Jamie Hamilton Smith. I'm 56 years old. I live in this complex and I go out to my day program two days a week – Monday, Tuesday. I'm having a go at the gym Wednesday.

A desire for a job in open employment

No. I feel sometimes I want to have a business – I used to have a job. I worked at AT. I wanted to do more – it make me feel – I want to change my lifestyle, and I want to have a proper job.

Health problems

I was 19 weeks. I was 19 weeks. When I was born.

Uh, my legs. And my back. And then my brain. And sometimes it's my speech. And sometimes it's as though I've been – it's hard for – I'm in a wheelchair. I want to walk. I want to walk and fix my legs. Doctors, they tried to fix my legs and my hip. I want to have a normal job. I want to do more and [my anxiety] stops me. And it's hard. I have a disability. And it's not easy. I want to have a normal life. I want to have a partner to help me and I want to have children one day. And it's not easy having a single life. It's not easy to have the single life. I want to get on with my life and not worry. I want to have a normal life without my mother, my parents.

Improving health by going to the gym

[The things that help in day-to-day life are] the staff. I go out and I'm doing some chores to help me. Doing my class. Keeping busy. [The gym] helps my muscles build because the muscles turned. My muscles turned very stiff and now the tablets I take – my muscles are losing the tone and my body isn't making … It's good for my heart.

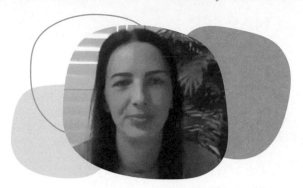

CHAPTER 3

Bonnie's story

My name is Bonnie. I'm a carer, but most importantly, a mother of a beautiful 16-year-old girl. She's had, and still has, multiple diagnoses, including progressive scoliosis, which she was diagnosed with at about 16 months old. She's undergone more operations and procedures than one could imagine, but has had 49 spinal operations and a lifetime of rehabilitation.

Burden and a pendulum of emotions

The struggles are all-encompassing. It's emotionally exhausting. Financially, it puts a really big pressure on the family unit. Very time-poor, your whole life becomes dedicated to these medical appointments. And there's a lot of sacrifices. And it's this big roller coaster of grief and loss, where you're constantly setting these rehabilitation goals. And you've got wins, and you've got losses. And it's just this pendulum going back and forth of so many emotions and so much trauma. It's a really difficult road.

Barriers of rehabilitation

I think the big one is the amount of clinicians we have in the rehab sector. And on top of that, it's a lack of having the right clinicians that have the knowledge for the specific disability, or for that ailment that requires rehab. There was a lot of disconnect between the public and private sector where she was operated on, and that referral into community. More often than not, there were links that we missed, which at times had the outcome of no rehab services unless I chased them up as her parent.

Carers are advocates in rehabilitation

I think the big one here is to continue to advocate for your loved one. Get connected, find support groups. Keep the goals during rehab realistic and orientated, not what the clinician thinks the goals should be. Stay informed, get copies of everything because sometimes, the connections aren't made and the documents aren't forwarded.

And probably, the biggest one is it's really fatiguing. So look after yourself. You can't pour from an empty vessel. And just know, despite how isolating it feels, you aren't alone.

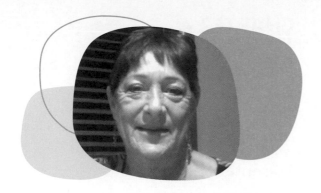

CHAPTER 3

Jacqueline's story

Undergoing rehabilitation

My name is Jacquie. I'm 65, and I've been very active for most of my life. But over the last few years, I developed osteoarthritis in my knees. Fortunately, I don't seem to have it in the hips. Eventually, it became so painful and so disabling that I went and had a bilateral total knee replacement.

Post-surgery – the rehabilitation journey begins

Rehab starts virtually the minute you hit the wards. They've got you moving and the physio comes in to visit you the same day.

A typical orthopaedic journey

It was really quite painful to start with. I was in hospital for about six days. Then I was able to go to a rehab centre where I stayed for another couple of weeks, because I'd had both knees done. I think the thing I learned about rehab most is that if you do what they tell you to do, even though you're a bit scared and you worry that it's going to hurt, it's okay. Every single lot of exercise that you do, you've got more movement at the end of that session, and you just feel better about yourself. I don't know that I would have pushed myself quite as hard as I needed to without actually making sure I had proper rehab. So, I'm very grateful to have had that.

Challenges and outcomes of rehabilitation

It was a little difficult to be away from my family for a while. And they missed me. Husband had to learn to cope on his own, but he's a grown-up, so that's fine. My kids are older; they've left home, so that was okay. But being in the rehab centre was actually worth missing my family. I had the 24-hour care that I needed. And they pushed me to get better. As a result, I'm moving around so much better than I did before the operation. I'm back doing most of the things that I used to do. You know, some things I'm just a bit too old to do these days. But I can walk. I can swim. I can jump. I can jog. It's just brilliant.

Take-home message

You need to understand how important the rehab is. I had a really good nurse that spoke to me very seriously and said surgery is about 60% of your recovery. The other 40% totally depends on you and what you do and the rehab, because surgery is only part of the solution. Doing the rehab means that you'll recover really well. And if you don't do it, you're creating problems for yourself. But if you do the rehab, you will be fine. You'll be absolutely amazed. Even though you do whinge about it quite a lot while you're doing it. But every day, it just gets better.

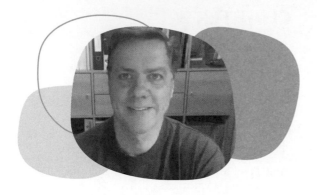

CHAPTER 4

Peter's story

I'm Peter. I live in the Blue Mountains west of Sydney, and I work at the University of Sydney, and I am married with four sons, and I was diagnosed with stage 4 lung cancer almost exactly two years ago.

Presentation of symptoms

I think my experience is probably a very common one in that you present for some medical attention with no idea that lung cancer is what's behind this thing, and I had been progressively feeling breathlessness, which I characterised as lack of fitness. Little did I realise just how crippled I was in a respiratory sense. So I thought, you know, I've really got to do something, I've got to see my doctor about this. There is something going on, and I ended up making a telehealth call and I spoke to a nurse, and I described my symptoms, which involved fairly noticeable congestion in the chest, lack of fitness, as I described it, and I think in her mind there was a real concern about a heart problem, and she said in a very unassuming way: 'Well, on the basis of what you've told me, I think this is a medical emergency, and we need to get an ambulance to take you to hospital.'

I almost couldn't believe what she was saying. Well, I think it's probably fair to say I didn't believe what she was saying, that it was a medical emergency. I was walking around, and I didn't have any pain, just had this congestion and really poor breathing. Anyway, I said, 'Look, no need to call an ambulance. My wife can take me up. We're about 10 minutes away from the hospital here in the Blue Mountains, and that's what I did. On that Thursday evening I went to the hospital, checked into Emergency. Fortunately, a very short wait time, and got to see a very outspoken doctor, who took the matter very seriously, and she made lots of inquiries and tests, obviously with a cardiac interest. And then eventually, I was sitting up in bed and had an x-ray done and that's when everything changed. They said, 'Ah well, there's quite a bit of fluid there on that lung and we're going to book you in for a CT scan to find out what's going on', and I remember the words so casually said: 'It could be congestive heart failure, or it could be cancer', which just seemed so absurd. But I couldn't bear the thought that she was right – and she was right, of course.

Diagnostic testing

After midnight I was checked in, and the next morning I had a CT scan, and confirmed that there was a substantial amount of fluid in my lungs, aand they decided to keep me in for about four days, and during that time I had a pleural tap done, which emptied the fluid on my left lung. It had to be done in a progressive manner, so that there wasn't a collapse, so over three days this tube in the side of my chest was draining pleural fluid to the amount of 3.7 litres from one lung, which honestly, when I look at a bottle of milk, I think: How did nearly two of those – a 2L bottle – fit in my chest that I didn't seem to notice.

So it was hugely shocking, and I was happy to have the interventions done, CT scan, everything. That pleural fluid was sent away for pathology testing, in the interim, and I was discharged, having had the draining done and the pathology tests initiated.

I went back to my GP. She prepared a referral to three different cancer teams in Sydney, and the first one that came back, I think it would have been about five days later, maybe more, was Chris O'Brien Lifehouse, and I had an appointment to go and see Professor Michael Boyer to find out what's going on. They had found by this stage evidence of adenocarcinoma in the pleural fluid, so we knew it was a cancer issue. Whether it was lung or something else was not exactly clear, and I remember being pretty alarmed reading that CT scan report. I remember thinking there's a lot of detail about what they're finding, but precious little conclusion, and that worried me.

I didn't know whether I should want it to be lung cancer or to be something else with a metastasis in my lung, I think it was all just so shocking. I reached no conclusion.

I remember going to meet Michael Boyer and him looking soberly over the report and saying that he wanted me to have a PET scan, which was a very typical kind of test to do here, and I'm saying to him, 'Well, that's very good, but I'm a bit worried that this pleural fluid might be continuing to build up because nothing has been done to deal with that. We don't know what it is, what's causing it.' And he said, 'Yes. Well, if that's bothering you, I tell you what, we'll send you downstairs and get a CT scan immediately and then we'll see whether the fluid level has increased since you were discharged.'

So I did that and I came back with the report, and I would say, within an hour I had had the test, and the report was done.

Treating symptoms

They had determined that there had been some increase in the fluid. So now I had the problem of continuing effusion, which is the fluid build-up in the pleural space, and the need for a PET scan to find out how extensive this cancer was, and he said to me, 'Well, you know what I think we might do is send you across the hall to the thoracic surgeon, Chris Kayo, and see if he can perform a pleurodesis, which would seal off the pleural space, prevent build-up of pleural fluid, and hopefully be the end of that symptom, if you can call it that. And I remember walking across, meeting yet another specialist and saying this is the situation – the story I've essentially just told you. He said, 'Yes, okay. Well, if you've got to have the PET scan, I think we need to have this done – the pleurodesis needs to be done after the PET scan. So I'm going to fast-track your PET scan!' And he said, 'We'll get that done at RPA. We'll get it done tomorrow,' and I remember his words: 'The man who does the PET scans there is the best in the state.' And so I was pretty encouraged by that, but not really realising what could be discovered with this test. Essentially, the test is looking for cells that are likely to be cancerous anywhere in the body.

Further investigations

So I proceeded to have that PET scan done and the test results were, I think, very encouraging. It showed clearly a tumour in the lung and a large number of very small nodules in the lymph nodes in the mediastinum; that is, the area between the lungs, and nothing else, critically no brain metastasis, no activity there. So this meant hopefully they could progress with the treatment, not having to consider dealing with metastases other than the lymph nodes. But at this stage still no diagnosis; adenocarcinoma but no detail on what it was. And one of the key questions, as you might expect with a lung cancer patient, was was I a smoker? Well, I was never a smoker. And that, as Michael explained to me, altered the likely diagnosis for me. It veered away from forms of lung cancer which were more typically associated with smoking, and to others, and the others had a higher level of treatability.

I was hoping that that would be the case. So from a PET scan I went to the pleurodesis which was interesting in itself. Firstly, Chris Kayo said, 'Oh, I can get that done for you at RPA in a couple of weeks' time', and I thought, Well, if that's the soonest, so be it, and then a light bulb went off, and he said, 'Or I can do it next Tuesday at Concord Hospital', and I thought sooner seems better than later. So, it makes no difference to me. Concord is actually slightly closer to home. So why not? Let's do that. What I didn't realise was that Chris had just begun a renewed thoracic surgery program at Concord. and I was to be his first patient there. I was hoping that he's not going to turn up at the operation and say, 'You know I want the such and such', and they say, 'We don't have that.'

Building trust

So there was a lot of trust required. But Chris was a man that I felt I could easily trust. He seemed extremely competent, and I thought I was in good hands. And so I was in Concord from the Monday evening, for about four days, I think, and the operation was successful, extremely successful and very painful, and I had a huge amount of painkillers of various sorts and they didn't seem to do a fantastic job, but I am sure that had I not had those, it would have been absolute agony. So again, I thought I came out on the right side of that equation.

And I had very interesting interactions with health staff and other patients there. There was one other person who was operated on straight after me, and he and I were the only two thoracic surgery patients in the gastric ward. And so came time to have my pleural drain removed, I had a crowd of nurses and other interested onlookers watching the process done by an RPA person, and I felt both a spectacle and very relieved that it was happening, and that hopefully the pain levels would go down. Well, everything went according to plan, and I was discharged with a relatively slow road to recovery.

So then, with another appointment with Michael Boyer, and then an update on whether there had been a diagnosis.

Receiving a diagnosis

In the interim, one test, an immunohistochemical test, was conducted and determined that I had what is generally called ALK-positive lung cancer, or anaplastic lymphoma kinase, which affects about 3 to 4% of non small-cell lung cancer patients, which is itself, the largest group of 85% of all lung cancers.

So there I was in this tiny little sliver on the pie chart of around about 3% of patients. They needed to get a second test before they would proceed with treatment because they needed to have the first test to verify it. So, a FISH test was conducted in a different way, and the FISH and immunohistochemical tests both indicated the ALK-positive diagnosis. And on the third of March I got that diagnosis, and was told that the treatment I was going to get was simply capsules taken twice a day every day, and that was it.

Targeted treatment

I was also told that that treatment had a limited effectiveness, and that at some point it was likely that I would need to change treatments. Here I am, two years next Friday, and I'm still on that original, what's called a targeted therapy treatment [Alectinib] which has some amazing effectiveness. So I was the luckiest. It's got some, as Michael would describe, trivial side effects, given the range of possible side effects of Alectinib, which can include, visual disturbances and all sorts of other things which are not good. I have got through this with really minimal annoying side effects, and largely am able to conduct my life as normal. With probably the biggest proviso being tiredness, probably from the treatment, and that's probably the most commonly reported side effect from the treatment. So it makes me not able to do as much as I could.

It [Alectinib] was first released to the public in 2015. It's the product of Japanese research and it has been on the PBS in Australia, I think, from 2019 or 2020, and that is a huge plus, because if I was in the position of having to pay for the treatment at the cost that the pharmaceutical company charges, I possibly would have run out of money by now. PBS sells it to me at less than 1% of the actual cost. It is extraordinary, and I'm extremely grateful for that – for the decision to put the Alectinib on the PBS.

Fear of progression

I think the biggest challenge is something that's in the background most of the time, and that is: when will this treatment fail? And will the next treatment be as effective? I know what the likely next treatment is, and the likely next treatment after that. And I know of the two drugs under clinical trial which are likely to be alternatives to that third treatment, or perhaps after that third treatment – they're nowhere near being available to the public yet. But I'm aware of what's going on, so fear that it will fail, fear of progression is what it is known as. Most of the time I'm not thinking about that, and every so often it grips me, and I just think what's gonna happen? What will the failure manifest as, and will a new treatment be as incredibly effective as the one that I'm on now, and you know there are certainly many anecdotal accounts, of having been on the treatment I'm on for five years, seven years, and there are accounts of people not enduring on this treatment; in fact, not enduring on any treatment and dying from this disease. So I can never forget the deadly ultimatum that it issues. But the range of responses is so wide and so generally optimistic that it helps me not be morbidly preoccupied with that. The other side effects really don't bother me at all.

Establishing priorities

I think what the overall effect of this treatment and sequence of treatment and likely trajectory, if you like, of my life, means I think about what my priorities should be; and should I be continuing to work as I am now? Should I be doing something else? And I think what's really surprised me, and this is so surprising because it's a positive, not just a relative positive, but an actual positive, that it has made me so excited to be involved in what's going on in lung cancer research, and what's going on with my fellow patients, and what sort of connection they need.

Incredibly effective treatment means that I can carry on. I don't have pain. I don't have anything that really strongly inhibits my activity. It's just the tiredness which I have to manage really well. So that's the limiting factors on my current circumstance.

Getting involved

The positive is what I indicated. I wish to do something that's of benefit to me and benefit to my fellow patients, and that's motivated me to get involved in lots of ways. I'm a member of the Thoracic Oncology of Australia TOGA [Thoracic Oncology Group of Australasia] that keeps me in touch with research initiatives. I attended the Australian Lung Cancer Conference just a week ago, and that brought me in contact with new patients. That's tremendously exciting when I'm able-bodied enough to be able to go there and learn and meet the people that are really the experts, the leading experts in Australia in this field. But you know there are statistics that I learned at the Australian Lung Cancer Conference which are really incredibly sobering. According to the Lung Foundation Australia in 2021, at least 37 people got a diagnosis of lung cancer every day and, of those 37, 20% of them will be alive in five years' time. So those statistics I just referred to are very significant at the public health level, and obviously for the individuals involved.

One of the world authorities on this lung cancer recently did a video describing ALK-positive patients under treatment as super survivors. So I've got reason to think that I'm going to be better off than most lung cancer patients. And I might just add that of the 20 or so patients that attended the Lung Cancer Conference, I think almost all of them were on a targeted therapy. That is a pharmaceutical treatment like I'm on and the latest generation of these therapies are allowing people to live the best life possible under these circumstances. That's incredible. And it's likely that this will be a growth area. So there's good reason to think that new patients, those 37 a day, will have a greater and greater chance of getting effective, enduring treatment. So that's tremendous.

Support services and resources

Pretty much anything that's been suggested to me, I've taken up. So I have been able to review a couple of publications for New South Wales Cancer Council, including a fairly significant publication on advanced cancer. So I don't have to be an expert in advanced cancer. I can just draw on my own experience, also to draw upon my critical observations of the experience of being a patient, and the information that comes to me. That's tremendous, because that's the sort of work that I really like to do.

But I'm also aware that at that conference there were 20-odd patients there. That's less than one day's diagnosis turning up, and I don't mean that the others have declined to turn up. A lot of them don't think about that as an opportunity, and some of them are going to be so unwell that it really isn't an opportunity. It's just something they couldn't reasonably do. But there'll be a large group in the middle who are sufficiently well to be able to get value from turning up at a conference like that, and also have an input into what the Lung Foundation in this case and governments generally are doing in relation to the lung cancer diagnosis and treatment. There's currently a big push towards screening initiatives, and that's really good. I'm more interested, I guess, at the other end of the spectrum. Not so much, how can patients represent their case to government and politics? That's highly relevant, but not the area I'm interested in.

Being a patient advocate

I'm interested in looking at how many other patients could benefit from the connections that I've made. That's really prompted me to look at forming a kind of register of patients who essentially would consent to being contacted by new patients, and being another arm of the support for those new patients.

And the way I'm envisaging it is that you would be able to find out who in your area has consented to be contacted to discuss the experience of being a patient. Who's got exactly your diagnosis? Who's had your diagnosis for the longest? Who's another man or woman, or whatever you want to meet? Who's a person of around my age, or younger or older? You can decide who is of interest to you, and the patients who sign up to be contacted do so willingly, and with consent and would be providing a limited kind of service. They're not a replacement in any way for the health practitioners. But they can say, yeah, that's what it was like for me, and it's really interesting to hear what it's like for you.

Specialist nursing care and support

I'm going to speak very much from the perspective of lung cancer, because at the moment the number of people that get a diagnosis of lung cancer today is approximately equal to the number of lung cancer nurses, specialist lung cancer nurses in Australia, so that's very small, and they might reasonably have a caseload of about 50 patients each. So after 50 days you've run out of space for those nurses to provide support, and I think the nurses' support is tremendously valuable, because the nurses can look at the whole situation of a patient's circumstance, not just the medical issues. They can look at how they are accessing and experiencing the medical services, questions that they've got, and that question of who else can I speak to that's got my disease, that's currently going to nurses. And that's where I'm seeing the next stage being available with a patient-powered project. Lung cancer nurses are tremendously good. There's recently, through support from Lung Foundation Australia, a program for increasing the number of lung cancer nurses. And I suspect this is a problem with very many serious illnesses, not enough specialist nursing care. And it's going to take, I think, some time for health budgets to adjust to that as something worthwhile, and I think I can say without exception, I haven't spoken to a patient who found that anything less than a perfect part of their lung cancer treatment experience. But there will be patients, I'm thinking, who are physically remote, in locations that are not at the doorstep of a service or of other patients, or they might be unfamiliar with ways of connecting to other patients in the manner that I'm connecting with you right now. So there's lots of opportunities to hear from those patients. And look at where there are gaps that could be filled with a service.

Identifying service gaps

The problem is fundamental. If a person as a patient doesn't take the initiative or can't find a means of talking about what their needs are, they're never going to be met. So we need to look at how we can provide a voice to those peripheral patients. …

I was on a panel at the conference, which included half patients and half practitioners. We were being just thrown some questions. One of the questions put to us was would we prefer to be called patients or consumers? I have to tell you I am so firmly on the patient side of this equation.

While I'm well enough, I want to be able to do as much as I can to improve the circumstances of patients who are most removed, most discouraged, I suppose, and my experience has been incredibly good. I know of other patients' experiences who have not been like that at all, and in that respect I have to be very careful that one patient's experience may say nothing about another's. So I'd really like to make sure that patients involved in this project that I'm hoping to get off the ground, realise the limitations. Their own experience may not be reflective of another patient's, but just having those various levels of engagement with oncologists, with radiologists, with nurses, and the other patients, all can contribute to an improved experience. So that's my goal.

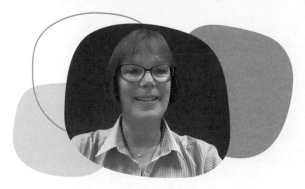

CHAPTER 4

Rebecca's story

My name is Rebecca Palmer. I'm a nurse practitioner for the Supportive and Palliative Care Service. I have been a registered nurse for over 30 years, and have worked in the area of palliative care for about the past 23 years. That role has encompassed hospice setting, the hospital, community and residential aged care as well.

I tried a number of avenues of looking into clinical and also management, and found that I was definitely much more of a clinician and much more of a hands-on clinician. And so I undertook my Masters in Nurse Practitioner through Sydney University. That course was incredibly challenging, but incredibly rewarding, as I was working full time in a transitional nurse position while studying part time as well.

The course ran over three years, and I graduated and became endorsed through the Nursing and Midwifery Board of Australia two years ago. So, my role as a nurse practitioner incorporates advanced care practice, and I also have skills that then allow me to do advanced practice, which incorporates pharmacology and also diagnostics.

The nurse practitioner role has four domains, which incorporate clinical, education, research and leadership. The role is predominantly about 80% clinical and 20% non-clinical, as in teaching and research.

Scope of practice

As a nurse practitioner, you develop a scope of practice which is very specific to you and your role that you do, and that is incorporated within the organisation that you work with, and the scope of practice usually is reviewed somewhere between every three to five years.

That's my current role. And I absolutely love my job. It's just really, really rewarding, and has been everything that I hoped it would be, and as it continues to grow over the years.

My role is predominantly based out in the community, which is where my passion lies for palliative care, and that incorporates being able to support people to stay at home for their end-of-life care or for them to remain at home for as long as possible. I also support residential aged-care facilities as well: I provide an in-reach service. We bring our specialist palliative care to residential aged-care facilities. I support the disability sector as well, and also have outpatient clinics that also provide a more equitable access to people in our more remote and rural areas of our local health district.

So that's my current role at the moment. Part of the role is to undertake research as well. So we've just received ethics [approval] for a research project to look at community nursing and providing spiritual care to people with fungating, malignant wounds. So yes, it's a very mixed and very varied role, and occasionally we also have paediatric, palliative-care patients. We work with the children's hospital paediatric palliative care team.

Goals of care conversations

I think, particularly in the area of supportive and palliative care, communication is paramount. Being able to meet patients and families when they are coming to our service having probably been on quite a trajectory, having lots of treatment, and we're now looking at comfort measures and best supportive care, being able to have those conversations about what that actually means to people, I think is really, really important. And I think also being able to communicate on different levels; for example, like we're doing on this particular platform, through virtual care, but also just those communication skills face to face, making sure that you're actually having the conversations with the right people as well, is really important, and to make sure that the language that you use is appropriate, and understanding that we're not using lots of medical jargon and things like that. I think, particularly within this area, it's really important to discuss people's goals of care and what's important to them. They now know that they have a life-limiting illness, but it's what does that time look like for them and what important goals need to be achieved. Are there certain procedures or things that they want or don't want? So, I guess it's sort of being able to have those conversations about what's important to people, and that's very individual. And I think that's our role as clinicians – to actually establish what that is, and to start those conversations with people.

We find that using the Advanced Care Planning tool is a really good way to start if people haven't had these conversations – and that is a booklet and a series of questions that help to have those conversations if people haven't thought about them.

Often, we find that people have got opinions on things, and they've probably talked about it through their life, but have never necessarily formalised it. They might have always said, 'If something happened to me, I don't want to be resuscitated', or 'I would hate to, you know, have a tube in my throat,' or whatever. Often, people and families have had those conversations, but not formally documented it. And so we find that using the Advanced Care Planning booklet is a way to actually get families starting to talk about it, but also for the individual to start really thinking about what's important to them. What kind of things would they be happy to have? What things are not appropriate in their disease trajectory? So that is a strong tool that we use, particularly early on. I like to bring it in, and I find it's a conversation that at times can evolve. It's not always: 'Here's the booklet. Just fill it in and bring it back'. Some of the questions in the booklet can be a little bit confronting for people, or they don't understand; you know, maybe what artificial feeding means and things like that. So, as a service, it's our role to talk about that, and to work through with families, and patients themselves, what that actually means.

A needs-based approach

One need we fill is to help them and support them to navigate the health system because that can be incredibly challenging and overwhelming, and particularly if stressed and fatigued and unwell, that can be a challenge. So that's definitely our role. I think it's being able to provide support, both emotionally and physically, and practically as well, along their disease trajectory, so having the conversations that are appropriate at that time. So that can be about where they would like to have their end-of-life care, if they have thought about that. If they haven't, to actually talk about what options are available in their local area. That allows the clinician to start planning ahead for those things; for example, if somebody wanted to have their end-of-life care at home, we know that we're going to need equipment, and, potentially, hospital beds, and GPs available to do expected-death-at-home forms and things like that. So, it kind of allows us to start preparing and planning ahead for those kind of things.

Also our role incorporates good symptom assessment and management of those symptoms, and having timely access to medications or appropriate management of those things in line with their goals of care. Those are the kind of things that we look at. We also try and encourage people to, if they want to, find out more about their conditions, or what the process is going to be, to make sure that they use reputable websites, and so we do promote organisations like Palliative Care Australia, Palliative Care NSW, those organisations have information on there for families, written in appropriate language. And it's about potential signs and symptoms that they may experience, but also what death looks like, as it's approaching. And what to do after death has occurred.

Talking about dying

So certainly that is the clinician's role, to kind of walk with people through that, and to guide them and to let them know what's potentially coming. We know symptom wise and how we manage that, but also what is normal? What is the normal part of dying? We try to normalise that, because I think, as a society, over time, it has changed. It's not as visible as it used to be. And often I like to ask people, particularly family members or the carers, have they actually had any experience of somebody dying in the past, because that can also bring into this particular scenario other emotions and experiences from that time. So it's important, I find, to actually know if people have seen somebody die before, and what that was like. Because, obviously, it is such an individual thing – dying – that no death is ever the same. And so it's being able to sort of talk through that, and talk through the experiences that they had.

Services and resources

One of the services that we've developed particularly to support more regional and remote areas is an outpatient clinic, which is a blended model which incorporates having the nurse practitioner actually in the clinic with the patient. And then we're using myVirtualCare, which is video conferencing telehealth to the consultant who's based down at the cancer care centre. Normally for patients for this particular area it's over a 200-kilometre round trip just to see the consultant. And so what we've found is that by bringing this clinic locally, we can still then do the physical examinations, we can still do the prescribing, anticipatory prescribing if needed, but it has saved the patients and family a phenomenal amount of time and travel. That's a new type of clinic for our service, and it has had some really positive impacts on people's lives. It then means that I've met people in the clinic when they're up and well, and still able to travel to an appointment. But as things change, and they're no longer able to come into the clinic, I then have the ability to be able to see them at home, and also, then to follow them through into hospital as well, if that's the case. So there's that really great continuity of care, and very much for supportive and palliative care, we like to have early referrals so that people get to know us, and we get to know them, and it just helps with planning and conversations, and we're not meeting people when it's sort of at a crisis point. So that is our ideal model. Obviously, resources and things can be challenging with that. And so we're certainly looking at having nurse-led clinics and nurse-led models of care. And I think that's where the nurse practitioner role can fit really quite nicely into that. So that's one of the things that we're doing like I touched on before, we've got that in-reach model into the residential aged-care facilities to provide that specialist palliative care service. And we're also doing what we call needs rounds in these facilities, where a facility will identify a number of patients, they use the SPICT tool, which is a tool that helps to identify somebody that maybe requires a referral for positive care. So they identify people that are then brought to a meeting with the specialist palliative-care team and members of that aged-care facility. And we basically discuss plans for those people, and then follow those up, so that's something else that we're adding. There's also some research coming out into the disability sector as well. So they're looking at palliative care in the disability sector. And also with the paediatrics and neonatals, they've just developed a new end-of-life tool kit as well, which is just being launched, which is a fabulous document, and resources particularly for clinicians who are not necessarily working in that specialist area.

Service models

Palliative care is definitely changing [from just being for cancer care] and certainly our service – we've now become supportive and palliative care, because obviously there's the end-stage heart failure, end-stage renal failure, dementia, palliative care as a service, and not able to actually, physically look after everybody who's dying. So our role is to provide a consultative role to the specialist, so that patients will actually stay with their teams, but we will provide that specialist input to them. So, we're definitely developing our consult service, and just, for example, the hospital consultation team work, I think their referrals have jumped something like 400%, it's just phenomenal. We are now running a whole team, which has consultants and advanced trainees and clinical nurse consultants and clinical nurse specialists. And we're reaching out into liver MDTs, we're doing respiratory, cardiology, aged care, and looking at developing a supportive model in paediatrics as well. So, I think that it will never take away from our specialist palliative care. But I think it's providing education and resources and support to other teams, so that they are able to do that.

[In terms of further developments or resourcing needed for the future] I think it's like everywhere at the moment, staffing shortages are everywhere, but if we look at palliative care, it is a multidisciplinary service: allied health colleagues, occupational therapists, physios, diversional therapists, bereavement, social work are all areas that need future growth in to be able to provide that holistic approach to people in our service. So, I think we've been fortunate. We've had funding allocated to us at the moment, and so we're starting to recruit into those positions, and they will be absolutely invaluable.

But I think we also need to be able to have positions that can travel out to our more remote and rural areas, because, at the moment, things are still quite centralised, and as we know, a lot of our patients soon cannot travel that distance. And so it's being able to have a service that is flexible to be able to go where the need is.

Self-care

One thing I haven't touched on is just how important self-care is when working within this space. I think it's just really really important that to be able to stay centred and to stay with people in this space that you actually look after yourself, and that the organisation or whoever you are working for respects that, and also it provides opportunities for debriefing or clinical supervision as well.

There's definitely people that will touch [you]. They may remind you of somebody you knew or your grandparents, or something like that, and I think it's just really important to be able to acknowledge that, and that if you find that somebody is staying with you when you leave work, that you're still carrying that person with you, that you need to be able to feel comfortable to talk to somebody about that. Because I think in order to be able to continue to do what we do, we need to be able to look after ourselves first, and to reach out to your managers, a close friend, or employee-assistance program, whatever it may be, just to keep you in that space so that you can continue to support the families and patients that we work with.

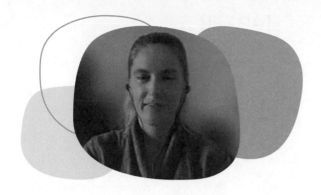

CHAPTER 5

Clare's story

ED is my clinical role. And so, we see everyone from all walks of life coming through there, a lot of them just with a background history of depression, others there because of their depression.

It really depends on why they're there. If they're there not because of their depression, then you quite often don't even recognise that they have depression, or they're being treated for it. But if you're treating someone with depression in the emergency department, it can be very rewarding when you see them go home and they're getting the help that they need. It can also be quite frustrating when you see them coming back regularly through the doors because they're just not getting that help that they require.

Challenges

I think sometimes, from an ED perspective, it's mainly the bed challenges of trying to get patients out of the emergency department and then into the beds. And quite often, you'll see patients, you know, 24, 48, even 72 hours later, still in the emergency department because there just aren't any beds for them.

Things that help

Our psychiatric liaison nurses are just brilliant. They're the best. And they're the ones that have the time to be able to spend talking and really dealing with the patients and the patients that need that extra help, whereas we can be going between someone having an MI, someone else having a stroke, and then someone with suicidal ideation and just not having the time. So definitely the psych liaison nurses.

Gaps in services

I think we could definitely do with more PLNs because there's just not enough of them to deal with the amount that we're seeing coming through the emergency department. Also, I think there needs to be more community help. I just think with the amount of revolving-door mental health patients in general that we see coming through, there's definitely a gap out there where there's just not enough assistance for them. They don't need to be hospitalised, but then they're not getting the help that they need out in the community to be able to stay at home.

Most important thing to know about depression

I would say that it comes in all different shapes and sizes. It is not a one glove fits all. So, I could have someone that's come in who's very depressed and very quiet, flat affect, all of that sort of stuff. But then you can also get someone that's also come in because of their depression, but they don't behave in the same manner. And so, taking your own kind of opinion of what depression should look like out of the picture also really helps, and just treating each person individually, rather than having a one-size-fits-all kind of approach like you can do with other medical conditions.

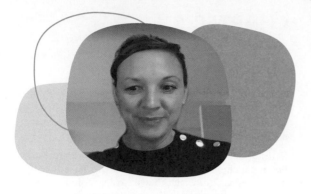

CHAPTER 5

Holly's story

I'm a community nurse, and I often visit people to provide all sorts of care, like wound care, catheter care, IV antibiotics, perform various assessments. These patients will often have multiple needs and are often living in really isolated conditions, which can often result in them getting depression. So, it's important that community nurses are able to identify the patients who are displaying these signs or are potentially at risk of developing depression in order to make sure that we intervene early.

It can be a bit of a challenge. A big part of our role involves providing education to the patients or clients. Often, people who've got depression will find it very difficult to engage with any new information or even have interest in taking on any new information. So, this can be quite frustrating with patients, especially if they require health-promotion education, because they've often got no interest in improving their lives or can see no point in making any changes. The benefit of being a community nurse is that we do get a bit more time with our patients, and we also have access to their family members and caregivers. So, over a period of time, you can often make a bigger difference by talking things through, offering different perspectives. And this can be really rewarding when you've worked collaboratively with other healthcare professionals and the patient's own GP. And then you'll start to see some improvements in the patient's mental health and wellbeing then. So yeah, a bit of a variety.

Challenges

I touched on a couple of things in that last question. Visiting patients with depression in their own home, although you do have more time with them, which can be a very positive thing, it can also be a challenge when the patient doesn't feel comfortable speaking in front of certain family members. Sometimes you get cultures or generations of people who will perceive depression as a sign of weakness, or maybe they just don't want to be a burden on people. So, they'll dismiss the idea of having depression and won't even acknowledge that their mood is low, for example. And they will often say that they're fine, and they will deflect their attention onto other people who they see as being worse off than they are. So that can make it really difficult to provide help and support.

Things that help

In the community, I've found identifying social groups that they might have an interest in is usually a good start, along with getting them to talk to their GP. Depending on their medical condition as well, there's lots of support groups. So, for example, if they've got Parkinson's disease or diabetes, there's loads of local groups, depending on where they live geographically. You can often tap into those support groups. Then they offer telephone services, internet resources, as well as the more face-to-face contact time. Even if the depression isn't linked to their medical condition, that can often be a really good place to start.

Gaps in services

I guess depending on the geographic location – there's not always something close enough by. And a lot of people rely on public transport or have not that much financial aid to get them to these places. So sometimes that can be an issue. And, also, just having that knowledge of what support services there are. So maybe it's more of a problem on the clinician's part if they're not educated or knowledgeable in those areas to be equipped to manage patients with depression. So that can also be a bit of a gap.

Most important thing to know about depression

I would say it's really important to be educated on the signs and the symptoms of depression, to have knowledge of the pharmacological and non-pharmacological methods of treating and managing it, and just having that ability to be able to talk openly about it with your patients, not being afraid of talking about depression as a topic.

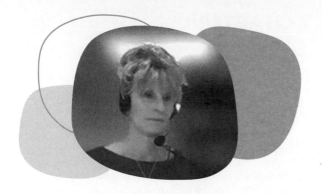

CHAPTER 5

Karen's story

I'm a nurse practitioner and I work with homeless people within the city and do clinics in environments where they go to get showered, or get food, and I see them for their medical problems.

It's very sad for them, especially when they're homeless. Most of their depression is not only the chemical imbalance in their brain, but a lot of it is due to environmental factors that are beyond their control. But certainly, I feel that when they come to see me, I always take time to talk to them, and that seems to help them quite a bit, talking to them about what they want in life, how they're going to get it, how they feel today, why they feel that way, and also, obviously, if they're on medications, make sure that those medications are working for them, and maybe adding something or taking something away, because they get really depressed to the point of, you know, it's the darkest days of their life.

Things that help

I think having had depression myself, I can relate to what they're going through. And having been in a similar situation myself when I was younger, I can very much relate to what's happening, and I can be very empathetic towards that. That really helps me. I draw on my past experiences to try and help them. And what helps me the most, what helps them, too, is when they come in and I haven't seen them for a while, and they're feeling so much better because either the medication's worked, they've been housed, or you know, circumstances beyond their control have been rectified, if you like.

Gaps in services

Yes 100%. To try and get a homeless person into mental health care services is extremely difficult in the city area where I worked because there's a lot of barriers out there for homeless people.

Most important thing to know about depression

It's to recognise at an early stage that there is depression going on, and to put a plan of care in place. And that doesn't have to be medications. That can be CBT, it can be anything that would help them to get over the depression, which, obviously, you can't just get over depression, it's a long haul. But what I found with myself was to make sure that I saw them as regularly as I could, so I would always book them in for another appointment the following week depending on where they were in their depression journey. I would give them then something that was constant. So I could listen to them, follow them, help them, obviously, with what I could with homelessness, and have that place where they can go where they feel safe, and they know me, and I'm not changed all the time. I'm the same person. And I found that a very good help.

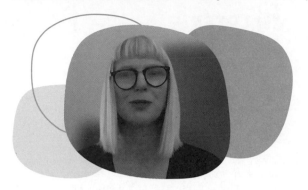

CHAPTER 6

Bronwen's story

My name's Bronwen. I'm one of two siblings, in fact. My brother Alistair [phonetic] is across in the UK, and [I'm] married to husband Stewart [phonetic]. And [I'm] currently residing at our family farm, which is actually close to my mum. I work for a global tech company, and have a responsibility across Asia-Pacific. So, my role is pretty full-on, and prior to moving back to Australia, my husband and I were across in Singapore. And due to to business that we were doing here, it was the call to come back to Australia, but also in where we landed was very much centred around Mum and Dad and them ageing and it being appropriate to be a little bit closer to them. So, here we are, just outside Toowoomba.

My mum, she was born in 1940, so 82 this year in July. And she's one of five siblings, and one of two still remaining. She has been a teacher for many years before retiring. So, she did approximately 40 years in the local Millmerran State School, and was a high-school teacher. She's a mum of two, as I mentioned, and her background has been highly educational. So, she's been a maths, English, history teacher through that period of time. She has been heavily involved in musicals with a couple of other colleagues of hers, which were the high-school musicals, and a prolific reader. You know, it was not uncommon to have Mum juggling at least two books. Maybe there was a third if she was getting a bit bored with something, and read for hours of an evening. And it was not uncommon to get up to go to the toilet at 2 a.m. and Mum's light was on. You know it's that kind of style. She loved to watch the game shows and she herself was in *Sale of the Century* and got as far as winning the cars. So, this is the kind of lady she is, right? And before Dad passed, she was living in the family home, and she continued to live there for a couple of years post that. However, currently, she is in Yallambee which is an acclaimed care, residential aged-care facility. And she's been there now for approximately 18 months, I guess. So, that's a little bit about us.

When dad passed, I guess when people have been together so long, they're a bit of a yin and a yang, right? And one will pick up the slack for the other and vice versa. And there was nothing evident before he passed away. And then when she was by herself we were here at that point, so we were visiting regularly and I'd pop in and sometimes work from Mum and Dad's or we'd be in contact over a weekend. So, there were just little things that started to become more noticeable, you know, forgetting bits and pieces, which, you know, that's not a big deal. We all forget things. So, you let those types of things ride a little. And then it would become items like food, for example, found in the freezer, or ice cream left on the bench, or ice cream left in the microwave because it's been in there to soften and then forgotten about. You know, she left the gas on, so we immediately decided to get the gas out and use induction in there, so there was no risk of the house burning down or her burning herself, etcetera. So, there were things that we were starting to do to just assist where there was – what we were finding was a little bit of a degrade in her level of attention to things like that. And at that point really, there was no labelling of 'Mum's got dementia'. It was just these things that are happening, until it did get to a point where I was noticing pills weren't being taken. She would have the Monday to Sunday pill pack from the chemist, and there'd be random selections missing. And it was like, 'This is not good because clearly we've taken Thursday's, but it's Sunday.' So, I was talking to Mum about that and initially it was, you know, 'Oh, I'm just being silly', you know? You know, 'I've mucked that up.' But then that became more frequent. And at this point, we had Blue Care coming in to fulfil some services for her because the family home has a massive yard. So, it was getting services to assist with the mowing and services to assist her with the vacuuming and changing of the bed and some of the heavier washing items just to get done to help support her. A little bit of social. So, they would go shopping to get in bits and pieces. So, it was a little bit of social, and a little bit of just supporting her day to day. So, we were leveraging what we could based on the assessment that she had had at the time.

And then things just started to get a little worse and worse to the point where she had hurt her back getting out of the pool for water aerobics. What you would seem a very simple thing, but that was quite debilitating for her. And then as we got scans and so on, it was showing a lot of degradation of her spinal … you know, little fractures and all sorts of little things that was the cause of that. And she got to the point where she actually couldn't get out of bed at one point. So, then she was hospitalised because of that. The pain got quite unmanageable. We had her at home at one point for around four weeks. And that was very demanding, physically and emotionally for both myself and my husband. So, we had done a – the word 'retreat' comes to mind, but that's not the right word. [Respite?] Respite. Thank you. Thank you, yes. So, she went to do a short-term of respite just to give us a little bit of a break. And then in various conversations we found that that was probably going to be the longer-term, the better, solution in order to help support Mum. And for us still to be very involved, but without a lot of the, well, emotional stress of being the number one caregiver. And the preference is certainly to be caregiver, but *daughter* as number 1. And as hard a decision as that is, I think it's been definitely the best.

Challenges

[The dual role of daughter and caregiver] is a little blurred I've got to say because one of the different things about the way that we interact with Mum versus a lot of the other residents who suffer dementia and various other conditions is that we do continue to involve Mum in lots of things. You know, we take her out of the residential facility for starters, whereas a lot of people don't tend to do that. And people aren't locked up, are they? It's a care facility to help support. It's not a jail and you're allowed leave. So, we just found that being able to have her removed from that environment and still socialise as she would have in her day-to-day life, it helps with some of the challenges, and I'll pivot back to those. But just to kind of highlight a little bit of a difference there, and for Mum – her attention span for things is really low. I mentioned earlier she was a prolific reader. Well, she doesn't read anymore. And if she's reading anything, it will often be me reading to her. You know, whether it's something on Facebook or if it's something in the paper or just something of interest, because she really struggles with that. And the challenge then being that she knows that that's a deficit for her and gets very frustrated with it. We're super fortunate that the frustration is not anger and there's no flailing of arms or screaming or anything. But she does get emotionally distressed about those types of things. So, I think that there's the challenge of just knowing that that's something can cause anxiety and being able to substitute that in some way. So, we also did try, for example, the audio books and things like that where she doesn't have to read, and it works for a period of time. So, it's certainly something that can help there.

I think, too, probably the greatest emotional challenge for me as daughter and as carer, is that when you see somebody who has had such a sharp mind, to struggle so heavily, that's distressing and it's working around that, but from her perspective, she has a bit of a reliance on me. Like I'm the kind of go-to, the bit of a security blanket I guess, and when she's forgetting things or she's feeling upset or it might be she's left the dining room and doesn't know how to get back to her room, something quite simple that she's done two, three times a day for the last 12-plus months, and she gets lost. So, I get the call and often it's a distress call, so it's just being able to kind of calm that down, taking some deep breaths and then, let's have a look at where you are, because we'll be able to find your way, you know? So, it's things like that that emotionally, I think for a lot of people, can be overwhelming and you really have to control the way that you speak to individuals and not make them feel like they're stupid. Because she'll say to me, 'Oh, I'm so silly.' And I'll go, 'No, you're not. We know you forget some things. See? That's perfectly fine. We'll just go over it again. It's okay. Don't stress about little things. That's okay.' So, you know that inside she knows herself that these things are wrong or 'I should know this', but often, it's not the case. And then other days, not a problem. Very calm. Knows where she's going and you sort of think, 'Oh, my Lordy', like, you know, 'Mum's back'.

You just have to take each day as it comes. And within a day, you can have good and bad times. She is certainly a lot better in the morning, and in the afternoon it tends to be the time – and they often refer to that as the sundowner stage. But it certainly is a time when she'll become more anxious and overcoming that is just talking through what's going to happen. And when she knows what's going to happen, things seem to feel a lot less stressful. And I'll often go and do happy hour in the afternoon with her in that period of sort of between 3 and 5, and generally carve out an hour there. And then everybody goes to dinner. So, there's a sequence of events that takes place, and that routine certainly helps – I think that coping and being a bit more familiar with what's going to happen. There is a lot of reinforcing that needs to go on.

Benefits of technology

Or even being available on the phone, that can help as well. Just to calm her down and I know the staff know that it's redirecting and it's reinforcing and they do a superb job. But then, she has an Apple Watch and that is one thing that she remembers how to do, is 'Hey, Siri. Call Bronwen.'

There would be no way that she would be able to operate a phone, and find my name and make a call. That would just – she struggles a lot with even making a note of, you know, if I'm saying, 'I'm coming in at half past ten. We're going to meet at this time. We're going to the hairdresser.' You know, jotting that little note down is a big effort.

Other helpful things

Certainly the watch has been a God-send because Mum did use an iPad for a while, but that became a little bit too convoluted. So, the watch has been great, and she also knows how to call Alistair, my brother. He's in the UK. So, she can take calls from him, and she can make calls out when she's reminded, you know, 'Give Alistair a call'. And I think having photos around are a great way to recall things. So, different events that we've been to, like my cousin's 70th, we travelled up to Mouramba. They've got a property up there. And there were lots of photos that were taken as a result of that, that we got developed. So, they're a hard copy, that she can flip through and we've written on the back if she's showing people, they can read and prompt her on certain things, because she's quite good once prompted. She can tell you a little bit about that. And the photos, we've got all sorts of family photos from different events, and Dad's photos and her grandkids and those types of things that she's got a recollection who, and is the talking point for anybody coming into her space, into her little unit. So, that certainly is good. And when she forgets where to go, when she sees the photos, 'Oh, yes, this is my space', because they're familiar to her. So, that would be another thing.

The reinforcing that I've mentioned, that is just a constant, and I find if I'm proactive with that, to say, for example, we use the little blue palm cards. They come in any colour. You know, just with lines, just a little palm card. And we write on every day of the week, and then we write what's going to happen on those days that I'm coming in. So, she knows when to expect me. But not just for her, also for the staff, because she'll often be asking them, 'When's Bronwen coming?' or 'Is Bronwen going to be here today?' or 'What's happening next?' You know, it'll be questions like that, where if they can see the little palm card, they can say, 'Oh, she's actually going to be in this afternoon', or 'Don't forget. You've got your hair appointment tomorrow, so you'll see Bronwen when she picks you up for the hair appointment.' So, it's a little thing, but now that everyone's familiar with it, including the staff, it's been quite a helpful little resource and reference point.

Being organised

You know, I'm super-fortunate with Stewart. Mum thinks the world of him, and he does a lot as a joint partner in this. It was a conscious decision to be physically here, and without his support, that would be certainly tricky. COVID put a twist on it and there's definitely a silver lining for me with COVID and being able to be working from home and be able to access Mum more easily because travel is a big, or had been a big part of my role. So, when that was happening, you know, Stuey was running Mum to various appointments, whether it's a dental appointment or to the doctor, or wherever she needed to be, and still does those things to help support me. So, yes, it does take a bit of organising, and a little bit of selflessness to do the things that you would do for a loved one, and just having to really step back sometimes to take a deep breath, because you can have the same questions over and over and over, and you need to answer it in the same positive upbeat manner, that you started. And sometimes that can be exhausting.

The most important aspect in the care and engagement

I think for me, and I guess this will differ for everyone, but for me, Mum was always part of the community. She's taught loads of people that are local. And so she's a pretty well-known individual. And so she has liked doing her afternoon teas and her lunches and being a bit of a social individual. So, for me, that engagement and not cutting that completely off, has been a very conscious decision to ensure that we take her to various places, and before the session started, I mentioned the Arts Council event that we went to just recently, where when people see Mum out, and typically it's with myself and/or myself and Stuey, my husband, when they see her out, it's almost a little bit of a surprise from people, which I find intriguing, right? 'Oh, how are you?' And 'how have you – you know, what's been happening?' which I find is perhaps not the best question because she struggles to respond to recalling that. But the fact that she's out and she's mixing with people, and mostly she remembers people's names or she'll say, 'I know that person. You know, who's that?' She just needs a little bit of assistance. Like she loves to just be part of it. And I think that for anyone who's caring for somebody, get them out and about, if you can. If it's not restricting them. She's got a wheely-walker, but she can still get around. And so, I say to her, 'You can still move, so let's move, and let's go do things.' We go to lunch. She has her standing hair appointment each week. So, she sees a different group of people there, and Natasha who she adores. We do an afternoon tea sometimes, where we're going out of the facility to do that. So, it takes effort certainly on our part to do that, because there is a bit of mucking around to get all of that signed off and okayed. But I think it's well worth the effort and, honestly, sometimes she won't remember. And you also have to go, 'Phew. Okay. So is she going to not remember each and every one of these events?' But I think what I'm learning is in the moment, she's enjoying it. And you can see that. When she comes out and she stays a Saturday night and she's here for the weekend, we've got Gorgeous George, the Maremma puppy, and we've got birds and cats and ducks and she's known the cats for years. So, it's some familiar things that give her joy and she'll have a glass of wine with me before dinner, and you know, it kind of, I think for her, feels somewhat normal, and what we would have done previously, you know? And just sit and chat. So, I think that's hugely important while they can, and while it's possible to be able to facilitate her getting out and about, that's what we'll do.

Benefits for you being Mum's carer

First and foremost, the residential care that the staff, etcetera, at Yallambee give her, gives a huge amount of peace of mind, just as I said at the onset, when there's things that are happening that really impact somebody's safety, you're worried, right? So, knowing that there's a bit of peace of mind that she's being cared for and the staff are great with her, and their understanding of her condition is really imperative. For me, that peace of mind is super. And the fact that I can still take her out and about, I think is super important. And we can have those little Mum and daughter catch-ups and she's got friends where we'll go for cheese and biscuits, if we're doing our happy hour outside of the facility. So, I think the benefit there is that you see her enjoying herself.

Services and support

Whilst Mum was still at home, certainly Blue Care, the support there was terrific. And I guess if we could have extended that, we may have been able to do that for a little longer. But I think things just kind of happened that we couldn't.

When they do the assessments, you are at a particular level, and so Mum's level only gave her a limited amount of time. We would use that time that some of the household-y things would be done, as well as a bit of the social outing and shopping and support to do those things. So, that kind of complemented what I was doing with her as well. But with somebody else, as opposed to just with me. So, that was quite good. And then when I was noticing that, with the pills, etcetera, then they were also popping in morning and evening to ensure that the appropriate dosage was being taken, because we're a little bit removed from where she was living at the time. So, that was good as well. So, we've had the geriatrician and the diagnosis and some of the support through guidance that he has given. We've had the informal information. Here we've got three family members, Sharon, her sister and partner, all of whom are involved in this area. And they've been tremendous. So, I think you need to source information from a variety of places. The internet, of course, is a great source of information as well. And now that she's at Yallambee, there's access to the paediatrician and the occupational therapist and you know, things like that. We'll get massage with the pain, and I sometimes take her externally to have that done as well. And we're yet to look at what dementia support services Australia have to offer. That's kind of my next port-of-call to just understand what can they do for support.

[In terms of using daycare services while she was still at home] Because she hadn't been formally diagnosed at that point, the short answer is no, I didn't. And some of the testing that is done by the geriatrician, Mum's a clever lady, right? So, there were some things that he's asking and she's answering, and I'm like, but this isn't a normal kind of recall. She knows some of those things, that's too easy. It's things that are happening – the here and the now and remembering those things that need to be done. And it took actually a little while before she was formally diagnosed. [Then followed respite service and transition to Yallambee] Because there were things that she was just unable to do, to go home and be self-sufficient. And that would have meant a full-time caring person to be with her. And it wasn't possible to have that really.

What interactions were there with health professionals earlier and could they have been more supportive?

Well, yes, maybe. It's sort of like rewinding the clock a little, isn't it? I think the one thing that I have found when you're looking for resources and services, it is really tricky to find the right place to get action, because even with Blue Care, there were a series of other assessments that were … Mum would be in months of wait to be assessed. Well, months is not helpful right now. And how do people fulfil that void when there's a need for care, to get a CAT assessment or whatever you need? There's a wait period, and that I felt was quite difficult because it's then finding, 'Well, where else do you go and how else do you best deal with that?' And certainly with Sharon and Michelle and Rachel, having access to them to help navigate that was tremendous.

And it will be interesting to see where Dementia Support Services Australia – what their recommendation might be for Mum in her circumstance. And now that she is in the residential care, whether or not that's viewed differently than if she was still at home, and being cared for in the home, as opposed to there, whereas I see that as her home during the day, but she still very much … we're trying to keep her quite active to be able to exit the facility and come and join us and do other things. So, you know, it will be interesting I guess.

What have you learned from your experience, or even hearing about the experiences of others?

Well, really only into my aunt who had been caring for her husband up until recently. And being able to sort of swap details and how she was handling certain things and what support that she was getting, albeit in another state, and sometimes state by state these things vary as well. But that was hugely beneficial to just know that there were similarities there and how she was coping with things that were sort of more advanced to where Mum was at that same point in time. Just to expect that or that these are other behaviours that you need to be looking out for, and just having somebody to talk to who can empathise with the situation really. But I'm not part of a particular group.

[Without other supports]

I definitely think that that would be imperative. You know, Lata was living with a full-time caregiver for a number of years. And I know she had a group that she would attend, and she found that extremely beneficial to be able to share what's happening and to understand more about why things were happening, and what she could do and how she could respond to that. I think it's probably a great idea for people who have access to that, to definitely seek it out.

Overall experience in summary

Like a roller-coaster ride, frankly. You're up, you're down. You expect the unexpected and just treat every moment in the moment, because there's lots of things you can't plan for, but those that you can, make the most of it and just ride that wave really, I think. There's just so many unpredictable elements and depending on Mum in particular on the day, as to what happens, or how she's reacting to certain things, so I think just, yes – be in the moment, and enjoy the time that you've got with these individuals. That's what I'd recommend.

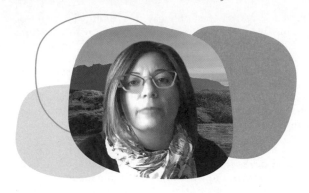

CHAPTER 6

Melissa's story

Dementia consultation and education

I work primarily as an occupational therapist and a dementia consultant to provide knowledge, skills and advice on matters relating to excellent dementia care for both clinical and non-clinical matters. And as part of that role, I've provided dementia-specific consultations and education services both within residential aged care facilities and in the private homes of people living with dementia. And I've provided and delivered assessments, managing cases, mentoring and modelling as well as environmental modifications, mainly to reduce the impact of challenging behaviours that the person living with dementia are experiencing because of their dementia. And to maintain their quality of life for the person living with dementia, as well as their carers who are living with them, particularly those who are living in the community home settings. So, a typical day would be me going into the person's home with someone living with dementia and, usually, their family are present. So, I would observe the initial environment – so, on my entrance, I'd look at the environment, just do a quick scan, then I'd ask some general and more specific questions about the general living situation. So, for example, who do they live with, what time of the day do you get up, what time is breakfast, things like that, just to get a picture of the person's day. And then I drill down into the day-to-day movements for somebody living with dementia on a specific or particular day.

And then, once all those questions were done, I'd get up with the person living with dementia and their family members and walk around the house and do a thorough observation of both the indoor environment and then go outdoors and do a more formal assessment of that environment. And whilst I'm scanning that environment, I would pick up cues for me to try to modify, and then, if I needed to, measure some steps or think about inserting or installing a grab rail, then I'd take some specific measurements for modifying the shower recess and then do those specific measurements.

Working with people in the residential aged care facilities

Usually, I'd get a referral from the aged care facility manager and so we meet up and I'd have a discussion with the manager and her care team or his care team, just to get an idea of what typical behaviours they were experiencing with a particular person living in the care environment. So, I'd get their perspective first. And then, I'd ask them what management strategies they have in place and then I'd tee up a time with the person living with dementia themselves to observe them in that environment, as well as their family members. Usually, a family member was available to join in the conversation, so I'd have a conversation with the person living with dementia as well as the family to get an idea of the likes and dislikes of the person.

So, really getting to know who the person is and finding out what their day-to-day movements were when they were living at home and what they liked and what they disliked to get a better picture so that I could feedback to the care home. So, it would have that type of conversation and then I'd go away and I'd put everything together trying to find things that the person living with dementia liked and what was the unmet need that the care home were missing usually. And it could have been something as easy as the person had a delirium or urinary tract infection and that hadn't been managed and that was causing the behaviour, or it could have been something more specific like the person didn't want to eat that fish because they didn't like fish. And so, they were serving the person fish and when they were serving it, they refused to eat it, and that was causing a behaviour. So, just things like that. You know, it's not that easy, it's not cut and dried. So, my recommendations were then made back to the care home, and then I'd follow up a week or two weeks later with the care home to see how those recommendations – one, were they implemented; and two, how successful. So, an evaluation of those modifications or implementations. And if that did work, then the case was closed. But if it didn't, then I would go back and look at what else was missing.

Importance of family members in evaluation

You know, I think they're very undervalued. Family members know the person better than anybody else. So, I think building those relationships with the family, getting to know who the person living with dementia was when they didn't have their dementia, is vitally important just so that we can be prepared to provide the best quality of care for that person living with dementia. Really getting to know the person and building those relationships with the family is vital.

Support and resources

I guess having an initial assessment whether that be the behaviours or the equipment or the environmental assessment. Those resources were a good screening tool for me to have. Also, having a template of a case management report so that I can compile a report for the care staff and the family members, knowing what resources were available to me in terms of mentoring. So, if I had to go back and I do an evaluation, I'd know what resources I could access from both where I was working and the dementia-specific consultation role that I had. They had a whole heap of resources that were useful and, obviously, education.

Healthcare professionals' education

So, my own education on current evidence-based practices and the education through my own learning through occupational therapy in dementia was a vital resource and I think getting to know the person is a valuable resource. So, the family members, we should tap into them more often.

After I graduated from my occupational therapy role, I worked immediately in a residential aged care facility for about 15 years. And that particular residential aged care facility had a dementia-specific unit and most of my time was spent in that unit. So, I think hands-on experience is very worthwhile. I think I've learned lots from being physically present within that environment and to see what the day-to-day living arrangement is for someone living with dementia, what conditions the care staff are working under, the challenges of trying to provide quality care for somebody against shortages of staff and time limits. It gives you a better perspective of how to provide those recommendations for people, particularly with living in residential aged care facilities. So, I think most of my experience has been hands-on and being around a group of other health professionals working towards a similar goal helps as well. We learned off each other, that collaborative kind of both education and coming together, sharing resources about specific people living with dementia.

Getting to meet a lot of people and networking is important, particularly with the dynamic nature of dementia. It changes so rapidly and it's so different for everybody and it's so different from day to day. So, really developing relationships with those that you're caring for and working with, building networks helps you to make a difference when trying to develop these strategies to prevent or to reduce the behaviours. Also, I have an educating role so I'm able to bring my experiences and educate people who are working looking after people living with dementia. So that's a benefit to not only myself, it makes me feel good about myself, but it helps others who are in those caring roles and trying to help them to be aware of these changes as well as trying to implement strategies, and be aware of these things that they could be looking out for when they're dealing with people living with dementia.

Best way for health professionals to support people living with dementia

I think having a thorough understanding really, not from a neurological anatomy side of the dementia and what's happening in the brain, but more so about what that person may be experiencing as a result of those changes in the brain. I definitely think that we need more education for health professionals, particularly GPs, because I think they are our first call of health professional that people will go and see when they notice that something is not right or that they have memory problems. So, I think, you know, upskilling GPs and with the education and not being afraid of exploring a possible dementia diagnosis. I also think support for post-diagnostic supports need to be improved. So, once someone has a diagnosis of dementia, where do they go? How do they access information? Who is available to help them along this pathway? And I think also from a government perspective that there needs to be a lot to be – to increase the capacity and the numbers of people working within the care environment to support those living with dementia as well as their families.

I think we have the education to provide information for health professionals. I mean, we've got organisations like Dementia Australia who provide a huge amount of education. It's a matter of getting it out there and outreaching people, and you've got all those complexities about rural and rural areas, cold populations, Aboriginal Indigenous populations, disability sectors. There's a huge variety of scope that I think we need to look at. They're not immune to developing dementia. So, I think there's professionals out there – it's a matter of bringing them all together and working collaboratively for dementia education and the intricacies of dealing with dementia for a wide population.

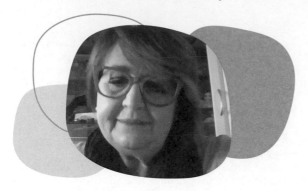

CHAPTER 6

Nell's story

I live in beautiful Port Macquarie on the mid north coast in New South Wales. I live with my husband and son and our gorgeous little toy poodle, Sassy. We have lived in Port since 2008, and I have really no family here. My daughter lives in Melbourne, and pretty much all my friends walked out once I was diagnosed with dementia. So in formal supports, I have none. And all family and friends live away, 10 to 12 hours away. Pretty much it's just my husband and my son and his girlfriend. And my support workers. So that's our little community that I live in.

Receiving a diagnosis of dementia

I have younger onset Alzheimer's. I was diagnosed in February 2020 after four years of fighting for a diagnosis. In 2016 I started showing signs of symptoms of dementia. And doctors put it down to stress. Oh, it's stress. I have worked in disabilities for 30 years, 30 plus years. I have been a disability support worker. I train and an assessor[inaudible]. My favourite subject to teach being dementia, surprise, surprise. So I felt like I had some insight into the signs and symptoms of dementia. And so I was seeing what I felt I knew. I wasn't remembering what I was teaching in books. I was driving places and not knowing where I was going. I was forgetting where I was going. Students had asked me to recount stories of my work life, and I couldn't remember the stories to tell them back again. I was forgetting names and places and couldn't follow conversations. Seeing things but not realising I was calling things by different names like dishwashers, calling them microwaves, and asking my son to put my dishes in – I meant the sink, but I was saying put it in the fridge. So all those sorts of things were happening, and I would go and tell the doctors all these things. And they would just say, oh, it's stress. So this all happened for pretty much four years. And it was very frustrating. I saw different doctors. They still would all say the same thing. It was very frustrating, and eventually after four years, I was finally sent to a geriatrician who finally did diagnose me with a mild cognitive impairment, which then went to a diagnosis of Alzheimer's in 2020, early, so February 2020. By the end of 2020, by December 2020, I had a cognitive driving assessment, and I failed it and had to hand my licence in. It's not bad for somebody who had spent the last four years with stress.

They were all my regular GPs. So my regular GP, when they didn't listen to me, I went, okay, well, I'm now going to another GP. So, I then moved to another GP, and I was with that GP for two years, and then in the meantime I'd been to another couple. And then finally I just wanted to see a geriatrician. I wanted to be referred to a geriatrician. So it was at my insistence that it occurred. Because I felt I had to fight for this diagnosis, I suppose, because I truly believed that something wasn't right because I knew in my brain that something was not right because it was too obvious. The signs were too obvious. For me having worked in the field, having worked with dementia clients, it just was not right. Yeah, the signs were there.

This is what frustrates me, and this is why I am such an advocator for diagnosis and dementia pathways from diagnosis, because I think what interventions could I have had in those previous four years that could have assisted me, such as medications? Like I have been on Aricept ever since diagnosis. I could have been on that back in 2016. That could potentially have been so helpful to me, rather than me going through such turmoil for four years. So would I be this far, you know, in 12 months from the beginning of 2020 to the end of 2020, where I actually had to hand in my licence?

And I no longer was able to work anymore because my memory was pretty gone. I couldn't remember routine. So I was no longer able to work in our business. I couldn't remember client routines. I could no longer do the rosters in our business because we have a disability service. So I couldn't do the rosters. I couldn't do so many things in our business. So being able to organise my executive functions was slowly just degrading and declining, and my ability to relate to people and my social skills, my filter was going, and my ability to relate to people and follow conversations and multitask, were just declining so rapidly. And my fatigue levels, and I was developing excess saliva, which I struggle quite a lot with. And you know, the medical fraternity has just been unable to explain any of that. 'Oh, I don't know, I don't know why you have that. You know, that generally happens later.' Well, it may generally happen later, but it's happening for me right now. So, everybody is an individual through this whole process.

And for me, this is what I really advocate, is that everybody who has any form of dementia is an individual, and their journey is very individual. And what happens for me will be very different to what will happen for the next person. So, I have swallowing issues. I have dysphagia, and everything for me at this point in time is cut up, is bite-sized, is soft. I drink from either a spout mug or from a straw. I live my best life, in the best possible way with my dementia. It doesn't rule me. It comes along with me for the ride, and that's how I decided to live with dementia, because so many of us think, oh, I have dementia, now it's going to take over my life. Well, I decided it wasn't going to take over my life. It was going to come along for the ride. And I was going to live well with it. But it certainly has its challenges.

Challenges of living with dementia

I think friends don't know what to do. I think it's kind of like the C word, cancer. It's the D word. It's dementia. 'What is it? D… dementia. You're going to die.' Yeah. I am going to die. I am going to die sooner than everybody else, but it is okay. I think we don't have the knowledge or the education. So many people don't have the knowledge and the education. They don't want to talk about it. I'm really big on talking and educating and sharing experiences. I already have my advanced care plan done. I have my will sorted. I love to educate people about dementia and Alzheimer's and living well with it and moving forward and how families manage and cope, because not all families do cope. Relationships change. The relationship you have with your loved ones may change, and you have to be prepared for that.

Some people come on board with your journey; some people do not. Sometimes you have to travel that journey on your own, and it can be tough on your own. But sometimes it takes some people a little while to grieve the loss of their loved one, because you do become a different person when you get dementia because your mind is different. When you have dementia your mind becomes a different world, and I always talk about my world and the normal world. And I do that in parentheses because it is a different world, and to begin to understand my world, you have to get into my world, and to get into my mind and understand where I am coming from and get into the mind of people with dementia to understand us. Because all of a sudden, we see things very differently. And our mind is confused. We've got lots going on inside it. There is just a multitude of things that's happening in a person's mind with dementia. So our ability to think, maintain thought processes, and do all the things that we once did, we now face so many challenges. And word finding can be difficult. Being able to follow a conversation. Just doing simple things now is so difficult. One thing at a time. Ask me a question, and then get me to answer. But please don't ask me three things and expect me to remember it all. In the past, that would never have been a problem. And so, families, trying to adjust to that, become frustrated. They become angry. You know, all of these things, you are not the person that you used to be, and families trying to adjust to that and your friends, they find it really hard to cope. So it's a big adjusting period. There's grief and loss for everybody, not just you, but for everybody. It's a great big time of change. And so, dementia is in itself not just an insidious disease, but it's a disease that affects everybody around you. And I think that's where people will count, because they just do not know how to handle it. And some people aren't good talkers and so if you're not a good talker, and you don't want to talk about it – 'I don't want to talk about that. I don't want to talk about death. I don't want to talk about dying. I don't want to talk about how things are going to be in the future.' They're out of here. They're gone.

I think I've met some really amazing people in my life. I had an amazing upbringing. I had amazing parents, who taught me amazing values. They taught me strength. They taught me that I was a beautiful person. I've faced death a lot in my time. I've had clients that I have held their hand when they've passed. So I've been honoured to hold people's hand when they've gone from this life to the next, when they've had nobody. I've just been really honoured to work in disabilities all my life and advocate for people. So for me, I have met and been at the lowest of the lows, and I've been at the highest of the highs. I believe it doesn't matter who you are or where you come from. We all come into this world with nothing, and we are all going to leave this world with absolutely nothing. I believe that death is to be embraced. We don't need to be scared of it. And I'm not scared of dying. I'm scared of how far I go with my dementia before I pass. I would prefer that I die before my dementia gets too bad. Because with Alzheimer's we know that you lose everything.

You forget how to eat. You forget how to drink. You forget how to do every bodily function. For me, that means I'm going to rely on my family to do absolutely everything for me, everything. With other forms of dementia, it isn't quite as crass as I say. It's not so debilitating. Alzheimer's is probably the worst one that you could probably get that's so debilitating. Of course, pick me. I got that one. And I guess for me, I hope that something else takes me out. You know, I get pneumonia or something before I actually have to go down that path of being totally humiliated, I guess, to that point.

Other challenges

Memory loss, I think, is probably one of the biggest challenges, memory loss, fatigue, and just community awareness of dementia. And I think dementia-friendly society is really huge. Doctors being knowledgeable on dementia in general, allied health. I have an amazing support team who are very dementia friendly. My OT, my speech, my dietitian. I've surrounded myself with dementia-friendly allied health, very dementia friendly, and they have educated themselves on that through me and through wanting to support me. For example, I have to go in for knee surgery, and I attended our local hospital just the other week. And I had to attend a clinic, and I went to the physiotherapist there. And all they are concerned about is my knee. And I said, yes, but I have Alzheimer's. 'Yes, well you need to be able to walk on a four-wheel walker, a wheelie walker, basically.' I said, yes, but I can't do that because I have Alzheimer's, and that's actually a trip hazard for me. And I can't use one of those because I trip on it. 'Well, yes, but you have to bring one of those in and use it because you can't come home from hospital unless you use one of those when you get your knee done.' And I said, I understand what you're saying, but I don't think you're listening to me. I said, I understand you're hearing me, but I don't think you're listening to me. I actually can't use one of those. I have Alzheimer's, and it's actually a WHS issue, and it's a trip hazard. 'Yes, yes, but you need …' and I looked at my support worker, and I said, she's not listening to me.

I said to her, do you not deal with comorbidities? 'No,' she said, 'we just look after the knee.'

I said, so what happened if someone came in here and they were obese or like what happens if someone came in here with another condition?

'Oh, well,' she said, 'we just look after the knee and what you need for your knee. We're not worried about anything else. We're just worried about the knee.' And I said how do you provide holistic care for somebody when they're going to have surgery? 'Oh, well,' she said, 'that's just how we do it in the hospital system.'

Interactions with healthcare professionals

[My experience with healthcare professionals so far] is absolutely appalling. Absolutely appalling. And this is what I talk about. There is absolutely no training, and I asked the pain-management nurse, I asked the physio, everywhere I go, I ask them, do you have any dementia training? Do you have any knowledge of dementia? And they go, 'oh, no, not really'. And then I say to them, so how many clients would you see, do you say, that would have a mild cognitive impairment, do you think? And they go, 'oh, we see heaps, because we see lots of old people.' And it's like – I rest my case.

Even when I go to, say, an optometrist or a hearing appointment or a physio or, you know, any allied health, they're all the same. I mean even the geriatrician, he sits there, and he goes, 'uh-huh. Hmm. Oh, okay. Right. Oh, I'm not sure about that.' You know, the only person that ever gives me any real feedback and someone that I feel really empowered by is a neuropsychologist. And so many other dementia advocates will say the same thing. Neuropsychologists are the only people that they ever feel empowered by and feel like their money is well spent. And worth her weight in gold.

Value of support networks

I do a lot of work with Dementia Australia. I do some research work with them. I speak at forums and webinars and tele-conferences. I also spoke to Parliament House with their dementia friends of something. Sorry. This is what Alzheimer's does to you. Yes. So, I spoke about the Royal Commission into – the Aged Care Royal Commission. I spoke to Parliament about that. I was very, very verbal about that. I had a lot to say. And then Forward with Dementia is another great organisation. They have an amazing website with great dementia pathways. Forward with Dementia. Another really great organisation is called Dementia Reframed, and that's with Gaynor Macdonald. That's another really, really good one as well. Gaynor does some amazing training, and they have workshops as well. I actually opened one of their – they have a thing called Charlie's Place. And I actually opened that down in – they have one down in Berrima, and I actually opened that earlier this year. And she also does a program called Gems, and it's an absolutely beautiful program, dementia program, and it's called Gems. And it's a beautiful way that describes the dementia states, and it describes them as gems, as gemstones. And it's a beautiful way to describe the states and how you see the states of dementia and the people in the states. And it's a beautiful one to do with families. And I've started it, and we're going to do it with my support workers and family. And I really love the way that it describes it and does it, and it's very heartwarming and beautiful. And it helps families see, I think, from my perspective. It's beautiful. It's by Teepa Snow, if you know Teepa Snow. And I really, really love the way it's done, and it's done very simplistically and beautifully. So they are three really beautiful organisations that I really, really, really love. But then you've got your dementia-friendly alliances in your local community that people can have a look and see if they're in their community. Dementia-friendly alliances are really beautiful because they're very community based, and they run locally. So they're really good. I'm currently doing an event called To Whom it May Concern. I'll be working with the Sydney Philharmonic Orchestra with a group of people, a group of dementia advocates, and we'll be performing down there at the Pier with the Sydney Symphony Orchestra on stage. And it'll be about our dementia stories. So I'm really looking forward to that.

Gaps

I just really want the pathway to be right. So from diagnosis, for every GP, geriatrician, wherever you are diagnosed, memory clinic, wherever, we have a clear pathway, so that you get your information, from diagnosis, you get information of where to from here. That's the gap.

Because generally you get diagnosed, and pretty much it's come back and see me in six months. I mean some people have even been told, well, you know, go home and get your life in order. That's not what we want to hear. On diagnosis, you need to be given some phone numbers, some information. Like someone has just told you, you have just been given a diagnosis of dementia, of whatever you've been given. What does that mean to somebody?

Like to me, I knew. But to someone who has no knowledge, what does a mild cognitive impairment mean? What does dementia mean? What does frontotemporal mean? What does, you know, what does any of that mean to anybody who has no idea? Then they go home and they google it. It can scare the pants off people.

Raising awareness

[Awareness is] poor. Absolutely. Yep. I mean the number one killer of men, the second leading cause of death in women in Australia, but what do we know about it? People are surprised every time I tell them that. They go, really? And I go, ah, yeah. Everybody knows about cancer. We all know about breast cancer. We know about prostate cancer. But what advertising do we see about dementia? We don't. We'll hear about, you know, on the news, you know, Royce Simmons has just been diagnosed with dementia. But we don't have any real advertising campaigns. We don't have any real advertising event for dementia. You know, like the McGrath Foundation has their pink ribbon event, but we have no real known event for dementia. And so, I just feel it's just no one has really grabbed the baton and run with it to go, hey, this is the number one killer, people, but we don't know about it. So, it's just like, ah, she'll be all right. It's that Australian attitude. You know, it's the invisible disease, because we all look well. It's not a good advertiser. You don't lose your hair. You don't look sick. We are invisible. It's just the brain's dying, you know. And that's what I say to people. You know, it's an internal, you know, our brain's dying, and that's the easiest way I can ever explain. You know, people go, 'well, what is it?' And I go, well, actually the brain's dying. It's shutting down, and they go, 'oh'. And I go, yeah. They go, 'oh okay'. And then you can see the cogs all of a sudden ticking. Oh, the brain's dying, like it's shutting down. And then you can all of a sudden see. And then people will say to me, 'yeah, but look at you. Like you remember lots.' And I go, yes, because that's stored in my long-term brain. You know, I can talk about all the stuff that I remember, but you get me to talk anybody yesterday or the day before, and it's gone. I will stutter. I will not be able to remember words, but you get me to talk about the stuff I know, and I can talk. But the minute you get me to talk about something I don't remember, my words are gone, and there I'll be. I'll be a blubbering mess. And it's bizarre.

Wishes for the future

My wishes for the future – that I cross everything off my bucket list. I'm writing some songs. So I need to get those finished. [laughter] So I can't die yet, because one of them is for my funeral. [laughter] So I certainly can't die yet. So I need to get that finished. My wishes are that, of course, we eventually find a cure for this insidious disease.

And I guess my wishes are that hopefully I have made just one small change and I've helped make a difference in some small, small way to somebody's life and helped them.

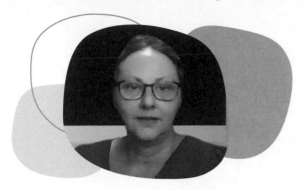

CHAPTER 7

Eleanor's story

Hello, my name is Eleanor. And in this chapter, you're going to read about my experiences as a carer. I'm a recently retired nurse academic. I trained and studied for many years to be a registered nurse and to be an academic.

Being a carer

Being a carer wasn't a position I applied for, wasn't a position I trained for. And that is the situation for many carers. Being a carer occurs suddenly as a result of a life crisis, be it a neurological event such as a stroke, a cardiac event, or any other medical condition, or an accident. People become carers for a variety of reasons. It's not a position they applied for or trained for.

Being a carer adds a different dimension to your life. It's another role. There are support services available for carers these days. I have lobbied and worked on many projects to get support for working carers. Life doesn't stop when you become a carer, life goes on. There are good days, there are bad days. There are plateaus and there are peaks. The rest of the world doesn't stop, so you make the most of it.

You gather people around you who can provide support for you when needed. You become very resilient, and you work out your own strategies to help you cope with various situations.

I hope you enjoy the chapter. And I'd like you to remember that when you're caring for people that there is always a significant other somewhere that you will need to support also. As the song says, 'Some days are diamonds, some days are stone.' I use a lot of music as a strategy for my support. Other people write poetry. They do exercise. They do other things.

So over time, you work out your own strategies that you need to support you as a carer. I don't have all the answers. I don't think there are any answers. And I could write numerous books on the skills required, the situations that you suddenly find yourself in. The sad times, the happy times, all unplanned for.

But they are part of life now as being a carer. After 23 years, I'm still learning. There are still things that I can learn – different ways that I can do things, different strategies that I can put in place. Learning never stops.

So, I hope you enjoy the chapter, and make a difference to your profession. Thank you.

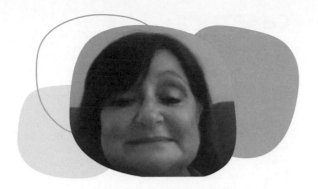

CHAPTER 8

Karen's story

Severe asthma

I'm Karen. I'm a very severe asthmatic. I've been an asthmatic since I was at least 19, though I had airway problems before that. I'm separated. I've got two adult children. And I am a very active person despite my diagnosis. I have many other diagnoses as well.

The experience of living with severe asthma

You can wake up to an amazing day, you can wake up to the day from hell where you can't even walk five metres, you can't dress yourself, you can't put your shoes and socks on. You need somebody to do it for you.

I've spent three months, five months in hospital. I've lost most of the last 10 years of my life from a virus that just sent my asthma into a tailspin. I've ended up having to have a bronchial thermoplasty in an effort to try and save my life and change my life. Fortunately, it worked and the last two years have been amazing.

Managing severe asthma

Changing your attitude. I don't usually try and say, 'I am an asthmatic.' I usually try and say, 'I have asthma.' So I don't identify with it so strongly. Also, exercising and taking control, working out the fact that I'm the one who makes the biggest difference. I exercise about six days a week, trying to make sure I keep my lungs as well as I can and the rest of me as well as I can, controlling my environment, controlling my diet, so I'm not eating things I'm allergic to. Anything *I* can do makes the difference.

Challenges of severe asthma

There are so many challenges. It's like losing control when you are so sick and being dependent on other people. I lost my career, I lost my finances. I lost so much due to severe asthma. You almost lose your sense of identity. You can lose just about everything to it. I put on weight. I couldn't even recognise myself due to the medications. It really is a tough road at times when you are living right on the edge at times.

Handy hints for healthcare professionals

I have amazing, amazing healthcare professionals. I love them, and my life has depended on them. The biggest thing I love them for is that they listen. And that's what I need from other doctors. When I have to go to new doctors, it's my biggest fear, is that they don't listen because my story is so complex, my medications are not standard. And often people tell me that I'm making mistakes, that my medications are wrong. And it's like, 'No, this is correct.' People need to understand that, often, we are very well educated about our conditions too. I need health professionals to listen to me, listen to how bad I am. Sometimes, I can fake it. I can fake it very well because I hate being that sick. So, I can turn up to a hospital appointment well made up, well dressed. I have driven myself, and I have literally 20% lung function. So sometimes, they can't prejudge what I look like. They have to really listen to me.

Advice from one person with severe asthma to another

Be in charge. You know, this is it, be educated. Educate yourself on every facet of your medication, know what your medications are, know what they do. Be aware of all of your triggers, and take control of it, and exercise. No matter how hard it is, exercise improves everything so much. I have improved my lung function out of sight, and I can do so much now. My respiratory team always says I'm the poster girl for having changed my life over the last two years after the bronchial thermoplasty. I have literally lifted weights, I have pedalled, I have walked. I kind of almost got into CrossFit. I box. I do everything I can. It is a hard slog. And some days, I am so breathless. You just want to give up. And you get COVID or you get the flu, and you feel like you've lost everything and you start over again. But you pick yourself up and you do it again. No matter how many times I get knocked down, I will get back up again.

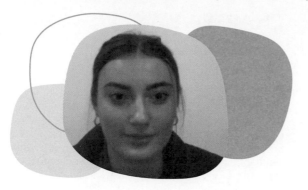

CHAPTER 8

Zoe's story

My main symptoms would be shortness of breath and chest tightness. It's kind of, like, I can't get enough air in my lungs or I can't breathe out completely. I get a wheeze, which can sound really bad sometimes. And then my symptoms kind of change with the seasons. So, in winter, my main symptom is a persistent cough. And it was really hard during the height of COVID as I couldn't really tell if my cough was asthma or potentially COVID.

I have very poor control of my asthma. Puffers don't really seem to work and my symptoms never actually really go away. I'm lucky that I remember all the steps of my asthma first aid, though.

The biggest challenge on me is probably the impact on my family and friends. Asthma is actually a huge burden, not only to me but those close to me as well. So, when my asthma isn't controlled, I'm not able to work, play sport, or go to family gatherings.

My GP is one person that I can't do without. It can be hard to get an appointment with them. But if I can't see my GP, telehealth is a fantastic service that you can use. And there's a hotline you can call, 1800 ASTHMA, where you can talk to an asthma educator.

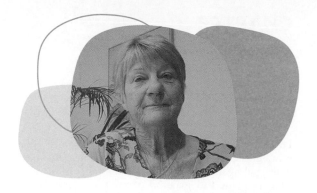

CHAPTER 9

Heather's story

Challenging times lasting several years

Well, my husband had a major heart attack, and that was one of many. He ended up getting a defibrillator and twice he had to go in for multiple bypasses. So we had quite a difficult time for a number of years.

I knew nothing about heart attacks and how you dealt with that and how you knew one was coming on in the first place. But in time I knew the symptoms and I could know when he was unwell. I had to do everything then around the house and worry about the shopping and whatnot and the mowing of lawns, all the jobs that he used to do.

Burden of responsibility

Well, I was lucky that he was an ex-sailor, and so we were covered financially by DVA, so I didn't have any financial problems. But I would have liked a bit of back-up in some regard for a bit of a break from him because he became quite obsessed with not being on his own. He was worried that something would happen if he was left by himself. He always wanted me around. I had family, and of course, they cared and they would drop in and visit and sometimes stay with him so that I could have a couple of hours out. But other than that, it was me doing everything.

Need for better understanding, guidance and preparation to cope with the overwhelming situation

I suppose these days there's respite care, which I wouldn't have known about back then. No one ever mentioned anything in that regard. Other than that, I think I would have liked to have been told more information about what was going on and what could happen because you're sort of in the dark a bit.

He ended up with a defibrillator, and more information on what could happen with that. When he first started having – I forget what they used to call them, when it would go off, it's the most frightening thing you've ever seen. And I think they call it a shower when he has more than one, and it would just lift him off the bed. It was the most terrifying thing I've ever had to deal with. So I think that sort of thing should be explained, that this could happen so you're aware of it.

Being heard and valued

I think give you more information on our level, not as a medical person, as a human being that's dealing with this problem and to listen to us. On a couple of occasions, I made comments that I was concerned about things, even to surgeons, and they made you feel like you're an idiot and didn't really take that you knew what was going on. But they forget that I'm with my husband 24/7. I can see changes. And I think they should listen to us because we do know what's going on. We mightn't have a medical degree but we can see that there's a problem going on. You know, take notice of us. We do know something that they don't see.

Reliance on and appreciation for the financial support

I was so lucky with the DVA. Someone would come out to the house and put rails up and all that. I don't know where I would have gone to get those sort of things done if I didn't have DVA so I don't know.

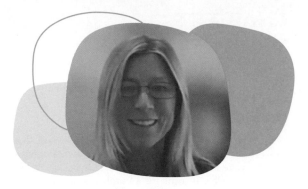

CHAPTER 9

Lois's story

Evolving career path as a cardiac nurse

Like any nursing career, maybe you intend to go one way and you end up going another. But I always worked in general medical, and I started doing that in the UK. And spent the vast majority of my time on a general medical ward. They upgraded the hospital, and my ward became a coronary care unit. So I naturally fell into that really. Whilst I was there, I did extra courses and then I just felt that the heart really is the heart of everything. I think if that starts going wrong, then everything else falls apart. So it just made me realise how important it is to look after your heart, and to be a nurse who helps look after hearts.

Passion for being part of the cardiac patients' journey and dedication to providing ongoing care

I also really like the journey from the beginning. You see these patients coming in in acute distress and terror, and even on the ward you see a real journey with the patient. And because care has become so much better over the years, I think it's such an honour as a nurse to see that journey where for the most part people do really well with the right care, and the right information and the right guidance. So they come into the hospital with a chest pain, and a heart attack, and you educate them pre. You see them through their angiogram and their treatment. You give them the education when they leave hospital, and I think at that point I started thinking: Well, what happens next? What happens to that person when they've gone home. As a nurse, you just say goodbye, and I found I was really interested to know what happened then, and luckily where I worked there in Wales, there was a cardiac rehab program, and I applied for a job, and then I could see the journey following hospital. And that's what I've done for the last 10 years now both in the UK, and after a few years I came to Australia, and I've been doing that actually, for maybe 13 years there, and I've done that for 10 years here in Australia. So they work slightly differently, but essentially the same. It's that aftercare and that education and that support that I think people really really need when they've had a cardiac event.

Commitment to guiding patients through their recovery journey

Seeing how good the treatment is, and believing in the treatment that's happening, and the development of that treatment over the years, I've been really privileged to see that progression. But also, I think, for a full recovery, you do all this hard work in the hospital, and if you want that good work to continue, I feel like you've got to continue supporting that patient when they leave hospital. I think it's imperative that they keep getting that support. So I guess in my mind it's just so important, and it's a real privilege then, to be able to guide these patients through their recovery, and to maintain and achieve a healthy life, even though they might not have been unhealthy prior. But obviously the majority have risk factors, and if you can help them change those and manage those, we can make such a difference in not seeing them again and helping them live longer and live a quality of life.

Challenges and barriers faced in cardiac rehabilitation

Firstly, it's a lack of belief in many that we, as cardiac rehabilitation specialists know are there. People aren't often referred to us or they go home, and everyone wipes their hands, and it's job done, on your way. So I think it's so important to get that referral in the first place. It's really good here where I work on the Central Coast. I think there's an excellent referral process, but I know it's not always the case in many parts of Sydney and Australia, and then the world thereafter. And so I'd say that's a challenge, and also people's knowledge about what cardiac rehab is – the general public, and that the hospital experience is very different from the after experience. I think people leave hospital with their drugs and their discharge summary, and then they just aren't followed up appropriately after that, so I think getting them while they're new in the hospital. Getting the referral, meeting them, in-reach is really important, seeing the person face to face while they're still in the hospital bed.

And of course we get referrals from other areas as well. That's not always the case that they're missed in the hospital. But I think that's one hurdle that logistically, too, our programs are often not provided out in the community where people live. We're always in a centre that they have to come to, and if they can't drive, or they are socio-economically deprived, or if they live rurally, there are some hurdles there for people.

Challenges faced by cardiac patients

That information, that they need to live a healthy life and avoid another cardiac event. I think just everyday stresses. The stress of everyday life and having to go to work, having to make a living, struggling to eat healthy, struggling to have the knowledge of how to manage their weight, their exercise, their physical activity, affording medications that they really need often, and the affordability of most things is a big issue now, especially now, and exercise people see as unaffordable sometimes, if they're looking at gyms and things like that, medications as I say and just getting the right information. There's a lot of social media. There's a lot of information out there on the web that isn't necessarily correct. And I think if people are googling the wrong thing, that can impact how they might recover effectively.

And I think, admitting maybe, that they have a heart problem. It's quite a challenge to admit that something's wrong with you, especially if you live a really healthy life. And it's because of a genetic predisposition. And so accepting that there's a problem and seeking the help initially, I think could be a hurdle for many.

Importance of recognising and accessing cardiac rehabilitation programs and resources

There's a lot online, but as far as we provide, from our Local Health authority, there is always a cardiac rehab program. There's normally one associated with every hospital, and unfortunately COVID happened, and a lot of services were disrupted, and I believe some or many are not back up and running now, which is a real shame. It's undervalued, I think, is the problem, by many health services, and it's not glamorous. It's not medicine. It's not promoted by a drug company so it's just not therefore provided. But if you can access it, cardiac rehab is shown in plenty of research to be really really effective in reducing your risk and prolonging your life and providing that support. So cardiac rehab, a traditional cardiac rehab program, I think, still in my experience works the best and online stuff and virtual stuff has definitely come into its own over COVID times, and it has a place. But I still feel like that face-to-face, that people-with-people situation, is probably more effective still, but certainly we can use our internet and our iPads and our phones now far more effectively, and people are more responsive to that. And of course we've got the Australian Heart Foundation that has a plethora of advice. I wouldn't say it's the easiest website to navigate for the normal, not-tech-savvy person. Even I struggle with it. There's lots of local facilities, there's all your surf clubs and your community centres. They often provide lots of information about physical fitness and diabetes support. You've just got to know where to look, probably. But there is plenty out there, but knowing where to look is important, and I think cardiac rehab, even if you don't come to a traditional program, can provide that. So I think if you're referred to us across the board, whether you're a STEMI, a non-STEMI, a valve replacement, a bypass, an elected stent, angina treatment, right from the GP to the practice nurse to the hospital, if you're referred to us, if they're aware of us, then we can definitely be your first port of call and point you in the right direction. So I really believe that's so important.

Cardiac nurses as health promoters and advocates for a healthy lifestyle

Starting with the basics, and just promoting health and a healthy lifestyle generally, we know that's where the bones of it are. For the most part, if you eat well and you're not overweight, if you exercise regularly, if you can avoid type 2 diabetes later in life and if you don't smoke, of course, if you don't drink heavily, and you know all of those lifestyle factors, as health promoters, I think all nurses can start there at the basics. No matter what ward you're on. It can come from anywhere to ask those questions. Do you exercise? Do you smoke? Have you ever considered giving up? Those sorts of pointed questions. Having the knowledge there, the nurses all have it, so just guiding any patient with whatever co-morbidity to a healthier lifestyle is really important. But it's easier said than done. I don't think any single one of us is 100% healthy. I know we all have our crosses to bear, but I think nurses in any area can promote a healthy lifestyle as regards to heart disease, unless of course, you're one of the unfortunate ones, whereby it is a genetic predisposition, and you have hyper-cholesterol and you're not aware. But looking at your family history, looking around your close relatives. What have they got wrong with them? What did they die of and knowing where to look is useful. But I think again as nurses we can provide that insight maybe, in any part of nursing.

Power of positivity, hope and patient empowerment in the context of cardiac care

I think it's a very frightening experience to come in as a cardiac patient into a hospital. And I think nurses, if they can get the basic knowledge of how well actually people do recover if they get the right treatment, and they do the right things. So to go at it from a very positive angle, which is quite hard when you're on the ward in an acute setting. But to go in there with always positivity and I think we're lucky in the cardiac world where we know that good treatment can really help, we know that it can be really effective. So, being positive and encouraging people to try their best to change their risk practice, believe in the treatment they're having, and giving up smoking if they have the stents, explaining to them the benefits of doing the right thing after they've left hospital. I think that nurses going into cardiac care are very fortunate insomuch as they can provide a really positive outlook for people, whereas I think people … maybe who have kidney failure, or are on dialysis. We know that maybe they're just waiting on a transplant which we know could potentially be unlikely. I think, with cardiac treatment, it's kind of always fixable, and I think, as cardiac nurses, if we can encourage people to be positive about their health and make those changes, that they can live a long and healthy life. So I think cardiac nurses have a real bonus, a bit of a bonus card, a real trump card to give their patients, because we can actually make a big difference. The patient themselves can really change things around, even if they have the genetic predisposition, and they're already exercising, and already slim, and they already don't drink, and they already don't smoke, and the fact that they've had that MI, it's terrible for them. But it's testament to their fitness that they've survived it half the time. So then, to carry on and encourage them to continue being the person they are, maybe with a tablet or two, it's really not the worst outcome.

CHAPTER 9

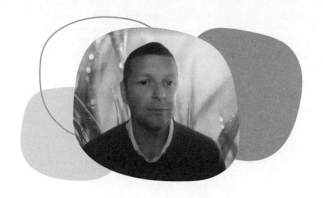

Nicholas's story

Personal background and lifestyle

I'm a 42-year-old male. I have 2 young children, a 6 year old and an 8 year old. I live in the central coast of New South Wales, and I've been here for nearly 8 years. I emigrated to Australia in 2008, just about to become a citizen as well.

I'm a pretty active person. I've played soccer since I could walk. I play various other sports. I also coach soccer at the moment, for my kids. I enjoy being outdoors at the beach, at the park, in the forest, wherever it is, being active the whole time. I'm a project manager for an engineering company and that keeps me stressed occasionally, but not constantly.

Discovering and confronting coronary heart disease

I was playing football in late September last year and I felt a pain in the centre of my chest, like a squeezing basically, which I initially put down to a cold that I'd had a couple of days previously, and thought maybe there's an infection or something, so I didn't think too much of it. And then the same thing happened. The next week I was playing soccer again, and I felt a squeezing, and it only came around when I was running. And when I stopped running, it went. But it was there constantly whilst I was running. And I realised that that wasn't linked to a cold or anything, and I needed to go and see my doctor, which I did. And after three or four weeks of various tests, including ECGs, blood samples, and finally a CT scan. And after the CT scan, I was called up. 'So we think we found a blockage. Please admit yourself to hospital.' Which was a surprise, to say the least.

Surprise and disbelief at being diagnosed with heart disease

I never expected that I would have heart disease. From what I know of the risk factors, I have none of them. There's no family history, I exercise, I eat well. I don't drink heavily. I don't smoke. So why was it happening to me? Perhaps stress might have had something to do with it. I'm going through a separation and divorce. So there's stresses on my life outside of the norm. But a lot of people are going through the same. So it was a total shock to find out that I had heart disease, and my left main artery was 70% blocked.

Available treatment options and their decision-making process

The blockage was confirmed on Friday the fourth of November in an angiogram and I was conscious through that. It's a minor procedure, so I was conscious. It hurt but I was aware, and the people doing it said, we found this blockage. You have two options to resolve it. We recommend option number one, which was bypass surgery. So full – open up the chest. We attach some arteries, veins, to basically go round the blockage, and option 2 was a stent to open up the current blockage. The reason they didn't recommend that was mainly because it's not a long-term permanent solution. So after 10 or so years you may need to have it done again, and given my age, because I'm early forties, I didn't really want to have to go through the same thing again at 52. So I was hoping that doing the bypass surgery would be the long-term once-and-done solution. So I made that choice fairly quickly with consultation from the doctors and surgeons at Gosford Hospital.

Journey through surgery, recovery and discharge

And over the weekend I had transport arranged, and a surgeon confirmed to do the operation at Royal North Shore Hospital. I was transferred there on Monday morning, Monday, the seventh of November, and I had the operation on the same day in the afternoon. So the surgery itself took approximately three, three-and-a-half hours from what I was told, I was unconscious. They opened me up, and, in fact, did a triple bypass, so there was an artery linked before the blockage to my heart. So bypass that, and there were two – well, one vein taken out of my leg and cut in half, and then put in as two fail safes. So it's a triple bypass, but all in one location. Realistically. I woke up in intensive care. I think I went into the surgery around about 1 o'clock in the afternoon. I woke up around 7–7.30. I had a tube down my throat. I was awake, but not really aware. I knew that I was in a lot of pain, and also I was on a lot of medication and just coming out of the anaesthetic. And I was able to have ice chips. That's the first thing I remember was someone said, 'Would you like some ice chips?', once the tube was out of my throat. 'Oh, ice chips sounds like the best thing ever. Yes, please.' And so I had some ice chips and basically I was in intensive care for 48 hours. Pretty much. Then I was able to move to a regular ward after that. So Wednesday afternoon I moved to a regular ward. I was in there for 48 hours, and I was actually able to get discharged on the Friday, which was really fast in terms of regular recovery time, but because I started from a reasonably fit base. I was young and competitive often, so I was trying to challenge myself to bounce back as best I could from this massive surgery, and when people say it feels like you've been hit by a truck, I've never been hit by a truck, but I definitely don't want to be based on what I experienced post surgery, because you're cut open. I was stitched together. I had lacerations in my leg where the vein came out. Another laceration where they went to get a vein, but couldn't find one, possibly because I already had a metal plate in my leg – previous soccer injury. And it was incredibly full on. But I was well cared for in the hospital for those days, and I felt strong enough in myself that when they said, 'Would you like to be discharged on the Friday?' It was yes, absolutely. I want to go back to where I live and recover there.

Physical limitations and challenges

There were multiple challenges. Being so used to being physically capable, I really couldn't do much else other than sit down and walk. Lying down was incredibly painful. It hurt my chest, everything hurt my chest, apart from sitting still and going for a walk didn't hurt my chest so much, but it hurt everything, because it was physically exerting. I came out on the Friday, on the Saturday I'd been told, just rest and relax, but do walking each day, because that gets your blood flowing, gets you breathing, keeps infections out of the lungs, and also starts to rebuild your physical capacity.

And the first walk I did was along the beach front at Ettalong, and I walked 100 metres and then I sat on a bench for about 20 minutes and then I walked the 100 metres back to the car, and I was absolutely pooped. It took everything I had to do that, and I was shattered basically – back to sitting down. That capacity increased as I walked every day for four weeks, basically, and in the first week, maybe I got up to 400 metres.

Other challenges were whenever you sat down or stood up, you weren't allowed to use your arms to push up or push down. So I had to keep my arms crossed because that would exert stress upon the centre of the chest and potentially compromise the healing.

And I couldn't do things like cooking, going to the shops and carrying things. Couldn't carry anything, washing, cleaning, all that kind of stuff.

Support network during the recovery process

I was very fortunate. I was assisted by my partner, Janet. A five-minute walk away from where I was living, was with me every day, came to see me in the hospital every day as well, just provided absolute fundamental support.

My parents flew over from the UK and spent four weeks essentially looking after me. I'm pretty sure I'll return the favour to them in the coming years. But it was amazing just that they said, 'We're thinking about coming over' when I told them I had to have the surgery, and I said, 'Well wait until afterwards, and I'll let you know'. But by the time I'd come out of surgery and I thought, actually, Yes, please, they'd already booked their flights, and were coming out, so I was supported by them and friends locally as well. A couple of friends, one in particular, a guy called Peter, made me food every day and brought it round. He was working locally-ish, but not necessarily right next to where I was at. He made me hearty meals that were wholesome and full of good healing stuff and brought it to me, and hung out with me and talked because everyone else is at work during this time, so I didn't have a huge amount of company other than my parents. So it was really nice to see him. That was my personal support network.

Importance of cardiac rehabilitation programs in supporting the recovery journey

I also was contacted through Woy Woy Hospital. They'd been given my details from Gosford Hospital, and they run a rehabilitation program there and invited me to attend. Basically, it was twice a week. Two hours, one hour of physical exercise and one hour of education, and I absolutely wanted to do that, because any opportunity to improve my recovery and get to the endpoint, as in being capable again, was absolutely welcomed, and they had a small team. But of the most lovely people who helped push me in really small increments to work on my physical abilities, and with things like treadmill, cycling, steps, rowing machine, and I started at a walk in week one, very slow walk on the treadmill. It was a six-week course, and we had Christmas in the middle, so I had two weeks off, but by the sixth week I was running a kilometre in five minutes again, from a point when, eight weeks earlier, I could only just about walk 200 metres.

Availability and importance of informational resources about heart disease

In terms of what I was provided, other than that support, there was also a whole raft of information. Flyers, leaflets, booklets. I got a blue book that was about 100 pages long before my surgery, in large print, so it wasn't a novel, but that had all the information about what was going to happen in the surgery, and what to expect post surgery. It was more aimed at slightly older people, but I could still understand from it what was going to happen in my procedure, and what I should be thinking about post procedure. And not just what I needed to do, but what other people needed to do, the support that I needed to have in place, and that was an incredibly useful resource, and I read it cover to cover several times before the operation and that really helped. I also got the education part of the rehabilitation program at Woy Woy Hospital which provided different information each week. So one week it was on food to eat, next week it was on physical exercise, then it was on something else, and covered a whole load of different areas, which wasn't brand new for me. I hadn't lived my life in a way that you would expect heart disease, but it was good to reaffirm that the things that I'm doing and the way that I'm living my life is okay and minimises those risk factors.

Quest for understanding the reasons behind their heart disease

Perhaps the one thing and this is incredibly difficult would be understanding why? Because I can't really put my finger on why I had heart disease. I know that I have been stressed over the last 18 months prior to the surgery. I also eat a lot of chocolate. A lot. But I asked that question, could eating a lot of chocolate have anything to do with it? And the answer was generally probably not. So it may just have been my genes, or bad luck, or something else. But understanding why it happened, if that were possible to determine, would be an incredible resource for anyone that's going through it.

Listening to one's body and taking action to maintain health

Primarily, if at any point you feel your body telling you something's not quite right, listen to it, because I didn't. At no point would I ever have thought I might have heart disease but I did. I'm so glad that I found out with time to have the surgery, no matter how hard that was, far easier than having a heart attack. Something that was preventable, because my body was telling me – check this out.

Gratitude towards the healthcare professionals

The only other thing to say is just a huge amount of gratitude to all of the doctors, nurses, surgeons, cardiologists, everyone involved at every stage was so amazing to deal with. In what is a life-threatening situation, the surgery that I had, I always felt cared for and safe at all points.

Ongoing processing and reflection

I've still got quite a lot of processing to do. I'm still going through divorce, and I kind of need to resolve that before I can then focus on this. But it has opened me up to the possibilities, and it's not necessarily a second chance at life. But it's actually 'Why, don't I make use of the time that I've got, because it is precious.' So there may well be some revelation that comes to me in a year's time that's opened my eyes. Yeah.

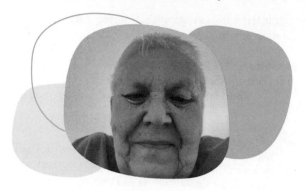

Sharon's story

Unexpected discovery of a heart problem

Well, I'm 75. I've been well all my life, really, and this was a bit of a shock. I had some chest pains and went off to hospital, they did ECGs and the various tests, and set me up for a scan. So I went home. Then I went back and had the scan. During all this time I had no chest pain, that was all gone, but I went back for the scan, and the cardio looked at it and said that I had quite a build-up of calcium there. So the only way to see whether there was any blockages or anything was via an angiogram. So I then participated in the angiogram, and they told me at the time that they'd put a stent in if needed – and it was needed. So they said they put a stent in while they did the angiogram and I haven't had a problem. I haven't had any chest pain since.

Challenges and setbacks during the recovery process

I did have an episode due to the medication that they put me on. The blood thinners. They sort of did something to the lining of my stomach apparently, and I was vomiting blood, and I had blood coming out of both ends. And yeah, so that was a bit of a shock. So I ended up back in hospital for another five days. I had three litres of blood administered to me there, and I had emergency surgery. But ever since then, everything came back really, really slowly. I was really slow, tired, lethargic, everything, no appetite. But then things started to come back slowly. My GP did a blood test, and I needed an iron infusion because my iron energies were really low. So I had that, and she said it'll probably take about three months to kick in which it did. And now I'm starting to feel I'm getting right back to me.

Unexpected health changes and challenges

I had no family history of heart disease on either side of my family, but my mum and my dad, my mum died from cancer at the age of 53, stomach cancer, and my dad had emphysema, which he blamed on the war, and he passed away at age 76. I developed high blood pressure. Probably always, all my life, my blood pressure has been excellent, but I developed high blood pressure. And my young sister was the same. We both had perfect blood pressure, but then, all of a sudden. Hmm! Both of us had a rise in our blood pressures.

Participation in a cardiac rehab program

I went to a cardiac rehab program, and that was the most beneficial thing I've done, that was really really good. We had an hour of talking. There were various talks about food, diet, exercise, your heart, and what it does and everything. And then, after that we had an hour of exercise, and the exercise was brilliant. You just do it at your own pace, and you start off with a warm-up, and then you just do everything at your own pace. You can use the bike, the treadmill, they have a rowing machine. It was really really beneficial, and I learned so much through that. I have a bike in the garage, an exercise bike, and I now and again jump on that, but mainly just walking.

Positive attitude and resilience

I have a fairly positive attitude. While I was down for the count she just took over everything. I look at the good side of it, sort of thing, and I thought, whatever it is, they'll fix it for me.

I didn't have a problem with the health professionals at all. Even when I went back into the hospital for that week after the complications, they were marvellous. They couldn't do enough for me. They helped me in the shower, they helped with everything. I think the health professionals probably don't get enough positive feedback, or whatever, but I think they're running their legs off. I think they're just doing fantastic.

Women to take their health seriously

Young or old, don't ignore any signs or symptoms, or anything, but call an ambulance because your care starts there. Don't put it off. Think of yourself for a change, and just get it checked out straight away. Don't wait. It's not worth it.

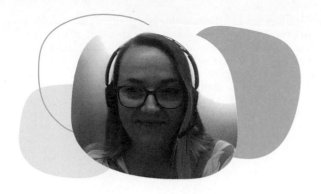

CHAPTER 10

Carla's story

I'm a renal social worker working with patients in the Hunter New England Local Health District's home and satellite services. I've worked in this role for the past six years. And I provide social work services to people who are in a pre-dialysis stage with their kidney disease, and also with people who are on dialysis treatment, either at home or in satellite units.

Challenges

Certainly one of the big challenges is their physical health. It's often complicated. There's often significant medical appointments and symptom burden. And this has a big effect on their quality of life, and that can fluctuate over their time on dialysis as well. Things could be going well for a while, and then a particular issue can really impact on them, such as a failure with their access for dialysis.

And as I mentioned, those symptom burdens – fatigue, and the other side effects that they can get. Their mental health – it's really common for people who have chronic health conditions to experience anxiety and depression. There's also significant aspects of grief and loss for people who are on dialysis and living with kidney disease – their loss of health, their loss of independence, their loss of future plans – and this has a really significant impact on their wellbeing. So I've found it's really important to support patients to manage their wellbeing and their mental health across all those stages of kidney disease.

Commencing on dialysis can be a really difficult time for people. It can be a really sudden and dramatic change in their life. It can be a struggle for some people to adjust. It might mean changes to their social situations. And some of those practical aspects of managing dialysis – the time that it takes to do dialysis, the travel, the financial impacts, the changes to the social situation, whether they're able to maintain work and keep working. So all that on top of possibly not feeling very well can be a really difficult time, commencing on dialysis for people. And it can take some time for them to adjust to that. I think I touched upon one of the other things that's come up a lot more lately when I'm talking to patients is their ability to maintain employment and work and the impacts on their financial situation. For people who are of working age, kidney disease, being unwell, starting on dialysis, can have really big impacts to what they're able to work or changes to their work. It might be changing to part-time or casual. It might be needing to find income support for the period that they're on dialysis. So, that can have a really big impact. And that can be further exacerbated by the level of support that they get from employers and family as well in that situation.

Services and support

I think one of the most significant supports that I see for a lot of our patients are their family and their carers. Their social situations are really significant supports to them. So I guess that's something to note, where we might meet people who don't have those supports well established, to be able to give them a bit more support in that situation. I mentioned about things like supportive employers. That can have a really significant impact for our patients. In terms of health-specific supports, our health system, our nursing staff with their education and treatment support, the Pre-dialysis Education program is a really significant aspect to facilitating people to be able to cope and adjust to dialysis and kidney disease. And I guess allied health services, such as social workers, occupational therapists, and dietitians are really integral supports that help people navigate some of those challenges of living with kidney disease and starting a dialysis treatment as well.

The other quite significant support there would be education and information services such as Kidney Australia. So lots of really good-quality resources they can access online to help learn about kidney disease and the management of it. But also things like the Big Red Kidney Bus that provides holiday dialysis. That's a really important support for people as well.

How a clinician can best support a patient through their journey

To sum it up, two things. Probably shared decision making, which is about working in collaboration with a patient and utilising really good communication skills. So, listening to the patient. Providing information and education to the patient in a language that they're comfortable with. Outlining the benefits and the risks that health treatments may have, or health-related decisions. Listening to the information that's provided by the patient's carer and their family. They often provide us with more information to be able to get a good understanding of this person's situation. And I think that's a really integral part of a way to support our patients through this facet of their healthcare journey. The other would be around utilising our allied health services. And I think we're very good at doing that. But in health care, we all come with our own expertise in different areas. We know that people's health has a really close relationship to their social environment – where they're born, where they live, their work, their age and the wider systems that they live in. Providing support across all of these areas can really enhance the patient's social and emotional functioning, which plays into their adjustment to living with a chronic health condition like kidney disease and having to start on treatment like dialysis.

CHAPTER 10

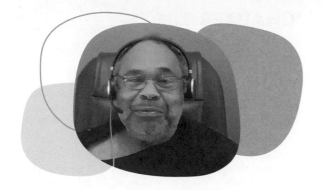

Dave's story

I first started dialysis back in 2013. About three, four years before that I was first admitted to hospital with all this fluid build-up in my body. It must have been about a couple of weeks in the hospital, I think in the ICU, just recovering and just getting rid of that excess fluid. And then not long after that, I had a biopsy on my kidneys to see if there were any issues. That's when I first learned that I did have kidney disease and there was renal failure.

And from there, it was just sort of trying to manage it as best as I could prior to commencing dialysis. Since starting dialysis, it's three days a week and in my situation, I do six hours every session but I think it depends on each person's medical health issues on how many hours they have to do to get a good clearance with the run. A few months before I started, I had an operation to get a fistula. I was lucky enough to get all that done first. I think you do need to sort of make changes and adjust your lifestyle, especially with dialysis. You get limitations on how much fluid you can drink. It's not just drinking water or having a cup of tea or just drinking soft drink or cordial. It's ice creams, custards, jellies, even like with fruits, the fluids that are in fruit. So you've got take into account anything that would have a fluid that would affect your daily limit.

With travel, even travelling, you can't sort of up and just go anywhere. You're sort of limited to places that can provide that away-from-home dialysis. You've got to look at where you can go, fill in forms, and that's pending a chair availability as well at the place – yeah, it's the availability – it can be done but you've got to really plan trips. I know people who have gone overseas or on cruise ships that can provide dialysis but it takes a lot of planning. You've got to watch out for foods. You've got to watch your phosphate, potassium, especially potassium foods because it affects your heart. Too much potassium can possibly kill a person so I think [that food has high] potassium like potatoes, grapefruit, bananas. Even dairy, I think milk, dairy foods have a lot of potassium. So, you really have to look at the food you eat. If you can't really take care of the fluids or watch the fluids in between your runs, it's the heart that can be affected after a while. And if you want to get on the transplant list, you want to make sure you can be OK on the operating table – your heart can take care of you while you're going through the transplant. You've got to look at the fluids and maintain that, stick to the limits that you're given to look after the heart while you're going through the dialysis. And looking at whether you want to travel down the transplant road or just maintain good health while you're on dialysis.

Challenges

Depending on the type of work a person does, they may have to leave work to do this. And that can also impact on a person's finances because they may not be able to enjoy the same lifestyle because they're not getting that same income they were prior to going on dialysis.

Distance – you know, do you own your own car? Can you drive yourself? Or even on dialysis, depending on each person's individual situation, some people can have a good run on dialysis but some people can come off [dialysis] feeling really drained and lethargic. And it might take them half or all of the next day just to feel better and recover and get ready for the next session. Their diet can affect that as well. Because if they're not eating the right foods and sticking to the fluid plans, that can also impact on how a person feels on the run, after the run, and prior to starting a session on dialysis.

Plus I think it depends where in Australia or the state people live, they may have to move to be able to do dialysis. If you're living in a country town or isolated area, you may have to move to the nearest major or central city, or big country town to be able to do dialysis. So, it may mean that they've got to move towns to get close to doing dialysis. [They might have to leave] their support network. So, like they may have a support network in the town but once they leave, it means they've got no support network there, at least for a while until they sort of find out where they're going. They might be able to build up a new support network with organisations. And even with the hospital that they're at, they've got people there that can put them in touch with new organisations that can help them and support them through their dialysis journey. But I'm sure a lot of people would like to have their family and friends around them, that type of support network.

But sometimes it's not a luxury for some people or it's not an option, if you're in an isolated town or community, you've got to uproot yourself. And even if you've got a family, you might uproot that immediate family like children, kids, partner. They might have to move with you or sometimes you may have to move first and they might have to come later on. And that way, it's a big, big change. For some people it can be a big adjustment, it can be challenging. But I'm sure if they've got a good support network there to help with that adjustment it can make it easier.

Resources and support

There are community support options. Like with myself here in the Hunter or like Macquarie, there's Hunter Primary Care. They can help with Indigenous people getting to and from dialysis. They can also help with specialist appointments. With like the payment, the consultation fee, they can help with paying that on behalf of the patient, the customer.

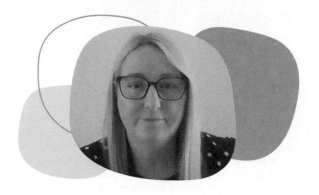

CHAPTER 10

Sarah's story

My name is Sarah Russo. I'm a nephrology nurse practitioner, and I work in a major tertiary hospital in a regional area that has inpatient dialysis as well as community-based dialysis.

I guess, to describe my role as the nurse practitioner, it is in the advanced nursing practice role. And what that actually entails is actually, for example, in the prescribing of the dialysis treatments, that would be the individualised reviewing of their blood results and actually, any issues such as hyperkalaemia. It is also looking at medications – that's reviewing and adjusting doses accordingly.

Challenges

The thing with end-stage kidney disease, we're talking about end-stage or just kidney disease, it's largely a silent disease. So often, symptoms don't really happen until about 75% of the nephron loss and/or kidney loss happens. So much like hypertension, often, there's really no symptoms until people find that the damage is done. So generally speaking, most of our patients have diabetes or hypertension, cardiovascular issues, etcetera. We need to take that into consideration, that those impacts alone are quite difficult to manage. Frailty is also a really big thing as well. We have an ageing population. Although, we also have patients that are much younger that are much frailer in presentation. So we don't really have patients that walk into dialysis from work and have dialysis. We're having a lot of patients that actually need to be wheelchaired or lifted with mobility aids to get them in and out of treatment. So that paints a picture of the cohort of patients that we look at these days. In terms of medical symptoms that burden is really in that later stage, particularly, in end stage where we start developing things – pruritus, renal itch, restless leg syndrome, nausea, taste changes, lethargy, poor appetite, sleep disturbance, etcetera. There are renal-specific symptom burdens that we need to manage, and that really impacts the quality of life of the patients. So that's really important that we manage those well. There's also surgical interventions. So in order to have dialysis treatments, there would be the need to go in and have a fissure created, or some vascular access put in place so that we can access a patient's blood. And there's complications that go with that too. There's hospital admissions, and issues around managing those important surgical interventions that happen on the way. And of course, because of their kidney disease, and also comorbidities, there is a risk of infection and sepsis, and particularly, when we're needing vascular access for the dialysis treatment. All those things are also quite a large burden for patients. And also, even transplantation in itself is a big surgical procedure, as well, that could be part of their journey. But mostly, it's dialysis-related complications, nutritional issues and dietary fluid restrictions, that can be really difficult and tricky for patients to work through day to day. And I guess, when we're thinking, not just medical, the psychosocial aspects are really important. Mental health is super important – that we address the issues as they come along. And this is life-changing.

And also, things like wanting to start a family and their sexual relationships and things that are heavily impacted. Becoming a parent may be much more tricky than what it would be for any other person. And so there is a very huge impact socially as well. And even for the elderly; for example, coming in for transplant, there are no services to support transport to and from dialysis. So being able to get themselves here and back, the costs that are associated with that and the organising around that is really complicated. I guess, the biggest thing, the dialysis treatment itself only does a very small proportion of what the kidneys should be doing. And so the treatment itself comes with side effects. So you may come in for your dialysis treatment to do a portion of what the kidney might do. But in actual fact, the reality is that the patients don't bounce out of here feeling fantastic. Often, they feel quite fatigued and not able to do much in the rest of the day or the following days. This happens three times a week, or more. And if you think about our dialysis sessions now, generally you would be coming in three times a week, and you could be just sitting on dialysis for six hours just for the treatment, let alone coming here and leaving. A full-day commitment. And when you think about the treatment itself, and all the complications that go with that, that's where we really look at the rest of the benefit of offering a treatment that may improve survival by a very short amount if it did. But really, quality of life for some people is much more important than actually the survival, having the dialysis. Dialysis itself is very different. Any other type of treatment is lifelong, and without it or the kidney transplant, life is very short.

Supporting patients

It's very important that we establish that therapeutic relationship early in the piece, that we take the time out of our busy days to sit and talk with our patients, and having really open and honest communication. Really explaining procedures and what's in front of them in easy language and terms that they understand. And using the teach-back method where you can talk to somebody about a procedure, for example, and you get them to explain it back to you so that you really have that two-way conversation and you know that that person really understands what's coming. And I think sometimes we are challenged with some really difficult conversations. So part of their journey, there'll be good times and bad times. It's really important to involve the family and carers as part of that shared decision making. And respect really comes down to understanding the goals of care. What is it that is acceptable for that person? And what is valuable and important? We talk about quality of life, so we want to offer the treatments that are in line with their personal feelings and their goals. So it really is the communication that's probably the key, and making the time in our busy days to sit and talk things out.

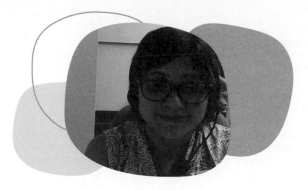

CHAPTER 10

Thida's story

My name is Thida Myint. I'm a nephrologist or kidney specialist working at John Hunter Hospital. In the multidisciplinary team, I'm one of the team members, as a lead in the clinical decision making as well. Because you can make decisions on when to treat, and how to treat, and when to discharge, and whatnot, in collaboration with the MDT team members. So that's my role as a clinician.

Challenges

I might see the patients for a long period of time, through the CKD stages. But they just go to dialysis, so they're about to change, right? That's where the discussion is all about, okay? So often, they will put me in the spotlight: 'Okay. I will do whatever you say'. Or sometimes, you will say to this patient, I would think dialysis may not be in the best interest, but they would like to be considered for the dialysis. So there will be to and fro of what my points are and what their concerns are, and then get to reach the consensus of the decision, like a shared decision making. So the other is when they go from the dialysis to have the donor transplant. But this is a transplant assessment, it's a process, but it's not a challenge. It's a challenge for the patients, but it's not a challenge for the clinician as such, but we've got to work the process through with them. Because it could be a long process. It could be a tedious process – do this investigation, do that investigation, and some of the patients get frustrated with that. So often, we can feel the frustration as well. Like, okay, get the cardiology clearance, get the whatever. There's a lot of steps in the process involved.

So as a clinician, in terms of day-to-day management, one of the challenges that we may often face is when we're going to dialyse this patient, whether in an acute setting or in a chronic setting. In a chronic setting, there's more discussion with the patient. Now you've got to this stage, what modality of the dialysis will be best for you – home-based or satellite-based dialysis? These are the sort of things that we would walk through. But in a hospital, acute setting, the patient may be very sick and unwell, and then you've got to decide what's best for the patient. Yes, you have that discussion with the patient, but sometimes the patient or the family may not have a good understanding of what's going on because the clinical situation itself could be very traumatic. So that will be when to give dialysis and what dose, and that will often be the challenges. So the other challenges that we could face will be when in a transplantation, because I look after the acute transplant patients as well. So you could have the offer of this kidney for our recipient, but then we've got to decide whether this kidney will be best for this patient. So when we decide, there is a team involved with a transplant, a surgical team, and a coordinator and whatnot. But often, this call could come in the middle of the night, like 3.00 a.m. So you just wake up and then, because you want to give the best-quality kidney for this patient, for any patient, but the deceased-donor kidneys, they are rare resources. And then, often, it might not be the best quality. It might be that the criteria might be a little bit extended out of what would be a standard kidney that we would see. And that's the challenges that we could face day to day in terms of the clinical decision making.

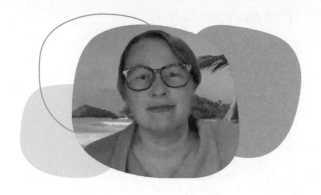

CHAPTER 11

Jane's story

Hi, my name is Jane and I am a person living with diabetes. I was diagnosed at the age of 11. So, I've been living with diabetes for about 40 years. I'm also a nurse, so I've looked after people who have diabetes and I am a nurse academic. So, I teach people about diabetes. I teach our future nursing workforce about diabetes and, hopefully, I impart some of the needs to have patient-centred care and to treat, maybe not differently, but to acknowledge that chronic illness is something that the person is really the expert of their own condition.

I've experienced using insulin in injections. I now have an insulin pump. More recently, I've been judged as a type 2 diabetic even though I have a pump and continuous glucose monitoring, which obviously wouldn't be the treatment for somebody who has type 2. But there is a perception that people of a certain age must be type 2. And maybe because I'm not a size 8, that also adds to the perception that I must be type 2 and it's diet and lifestyle related rather than the autoimmune condition. But I've had diabetes since the age of 11.

Struggle

I have to say that it was really difficult going through teenage and adolescence because I didn't want to appear different. And I guess I've struggled with that and struggled with the fact that I didn't want to be lesser or less able to do things than other people. And perhaps to my own detriment. When I first started nursing, I didn't want to have to be the one who always went for their break at the same time, even if it was really busy. The reality is that it would have been worse for me to have a hypo on the ward, but at the time, I didn't want to be a burden to anybody else.

I think what I would like people to know about diabetes is that it is that 24/7, 7 days a week condition that never goes away. And most of the time, I cope really well with it. If I come to you for help, if I seek help at an emergency department, it's because I need it. It's because I don't know what's going on. And I do worry a little that people aren't as up to speed with things like pumps and would not be able to look after me if I was unable to manage that side of my healthcare myself.

But really what you need to be thinking about, in terms of caring for someone who has diabetes, whether it is type 1, type 2 or gestational diabetes, is that it is a condition that people have to come to terms with. Gestational diabetes will last for the pregnancy but may become type 2 diabetes at some stage. So, there is still some coming to terms with that. Type 1 and type 2 diabetes – it is possible to have those and then become pregnant. And that again adds to complications. There's a change in management. It is quite difficult during pregnancy to maintain blood glucose. Your need for insulin changes quite drastically in pregnancy. So, it is difficult in that regard.

Judgement from people

I guess there's also the complications, the judgement from people. If they know that you have diabetes, that if you have a piece of cake, that you get that sly look, even though you know that you can now manage your diabetes and you can bolus with a pump, to eat virtually anything, really, it is still a perception that you're doing something wrong. If you don't tell people, then there is the risk that you are unwell and nobody knows what the problem is. So it's a trust thing, I guess. Trusting other people with your health information, with helping you manage things. So it is good to be able to have a trusted healthcare professional that you can talk to. And if you can be that for somebody, that's great. I guess the other thing is take an interest, take an interest in the person – how they are, what their life is like. And not just that they have diabetes.

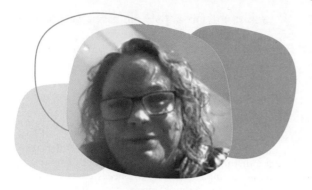

CHAPTER 11

Rebecca's story

Diagnosis

I was diagnosed in 1975, I was 18 months of age. And basically, I had started to lose a lot of weight. I was brought to my paediatrician's attention, but he basically said that due to my age, it can't be type 1 diabetes and he sent me on my merry way. And then six weeks later, I didn't wake up as I would normally wake up in the morning, and Mum's come in and she's noticed that I was out cold. I was in a coma, for which back then I was rushed to the Children's Hospital in Camperdown, and I was out to it for about three days. Another doctor's come in and given me insulin and within five hours I've come out of the coma.

I always have a vivid memory of waking up in the morning and seeing the saucepan on the oven, not on the oven, but on the stove and all the water was boiling because it was sterilising the glass needles back then as well. So as you know, they're plastic now, and it's one-time use and in the bin it goes, but back then … and she used to have to sharpen the needle on the brick. And you know, to me, as an 18-month-old, two-year-old, that knife was huge, you know. So, it was very vivid memories. But I would have to say that out of the years, the toughest years of living with diabetes was the adolescence. That was pretty rough because you wanted to be a normal teenager, but you couldn't be normal. You couldn't go out and be with the other mates and do what your other mates were doing. So that was a bit of a bummer. And I always say, man, if you can get through adolescence with diabetes, you're a strong person. You'll get there, you'll do it, you'll get to the end, no problem. It is a tough time. And I think also back in that generation, my mother was told that I'd probably die at the age of 40 and that I'll never have children. So there were all these negatives regarding diagnosis of diabetes back in the day. But again, as years go on and research and education and awareness, it's all just, it's better now. I'm not saying that it's not overwhelming, I'm not saying that it doesn't change your life, but in comparison to what we know now to what we didn't know back then, there's a huge change for the better. And of course, now we've got the tools such as pumps and continual glucose monitoring, and they certainly make the job of living with diabetes easier.

Changes

Back in the day, again, all those years ago, there was no such thing as human synthetic insulin. It was beef and pork. And man, they just threw the weight on you big time. You couldn't eat a lot of foods. I was called a junkie in Year Six because I was having needles and I had to look above that and not let that person lower me. So there was a lot of misunderstanding as to the understanding of what diabetes was.

So that needle situation ended up being from two a day, as you go into adolescence I was probably having – well, I was 'supposed to be having' four, five injections a day. So if you think about that over 20 years, that's a lot of needle pushing. It's a lot of holes coming out of your skin every time you drink a glass of water. But it's the body image as well that needles can – with scarring and dead tissue and all those wonderful lumps and bumps that we get over the years. Obviously, as a teenager, the way you look is quite significant. So these pumps basically have changed my life completely when living with diabetes. And I guess where the benefit is, is the fact that it's only 1 needle every 3 days now as opposed to 15 in 3 days. And I guess also with the fact that they're delivering at much smaller increments, so, whether you're doing exercise or whatever, at least then with a pump, it's a lot easier to manage. If you didn't want to eat, you didn't have to have your needles. If you did want to eat like a horse, that's cool, just tell the pump what you're eating. So there's a lot more flexibility with a pump basically doing it all automatically without much work. So there's a lot of burden in managing diabetes. There's a lot of headspace. You never get a day off. You're always thinking every five minutes of the day, what am I going to do now? What should I do now? Am I about to have a hypo? Maybe I'll get over a hyper. You just – your brain just doesn't stop. And that is where this technology is now, helping a lot of people because it's taking that thinking away and it's all doing it for you.

Important things for health professionals to know

I think they need to understand it's the headspace. As I said before, you don't get a day off and everybody has their own anxieties, whether you've got diabetes or not. And having anxiety about doing needles is not your ideal anxiety to have when you've got diabetes because that's really what's getting you through your life. But headspace would be my number one. But I think that's a very important thing for me, for up-and-coming health professionals to understand that, if you tell me to do something, I'm not going to do it. Don't tell me, maybe suggest, maybe guide, but let me make the decision as to how I'm going to do that and what's best for me. That's my feeling.

And everybody's lived a different life, nobody's the same. And I think they need to understand that too, that nobody likes to be told. Because of course, we're always going to turn around and say, 'You don't live with it, so you don't get it, so don't tell me what to do.' And we all say that, all people with type 1 say that, we're very precious in a way. But if there's a chronic disease that makes that individual independent, it's diabetes.

I think listening is a big thing. They need to listen because a lot of people with diabetes become very guarded as well because they feel like they're being judged. But they still need to be very careful as to how they present themselves or how they communicate themselves to a diabetic or a person with diabetes, I should say. Because, you know, we do pull that wall up and it's because of the fact that we're always sick of being judged whether we are good or bad. We never get rewarded.

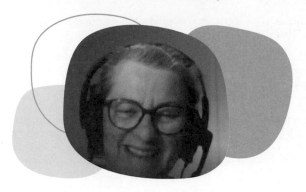

Ruth's story

There is no two days that are the same, in any way. And every single patient comes with a whole different problem to solve, or to work with, or a new challenge. So if you're looking for variety in your career, I recommend it really strongly.

And of course, the chronic care model is a really interesting way to work in nursing. Because you have to be holistic. You really have to look at the whole person, of what's going on and how, and working with people to problem solve. And I really enjoy doing that.

I describe a diagnosis of diabetes as like a newborn baby, which comes with its challenges, as most people can relate to. The difference with diabetes is the diabetes doesn't grow up at 18, and leave home, and hopefully go on to become an adult. So it never ever goes away. And I think many years ago, a colleague of mine was presenting, and she said diabetes is something that every morning (and this was some years ago now, so things have changed a little bit, but not a lot) but every morning, when somebody with diabetes wakes up, they have to think about their diabetes. I mean, some people don't, as we know, but to manage it and manage it well, it just doesn't go away. And I think that's one of the biggest challenges for everyone to understand – that we need to work with people while they try to incorporate diabetes as part of their life rather than it dictating their life.

We provide the medication, support, pathophysiology, our modes of management to new medications for type 2 medications, both injectable and non-injectable. And then, of course, newly diagnosed type 1s or people who have had type 1 for a long, long time, people who are wanting to become engaged more with technology in diabetes, people with quite severe complications from their diabetes. We also have gestational diabetes and diabetes in pregnancy. So people with type 1 and type 2 with diabetes. And yes, as I say to a lot of people, it's the booming industry without a doubt, and will keep me well employed into my retirement years.

It's really complex because people become very confused about type 1 and type 2. Someone in type 2 commences insulin and then they think they're type 1. Or of course, there's people who think they know about the the diabetes. Somebody might be louder. And they've got people judging them because people are saying, 'Oh, it's all lifestyle related.' People think that it's a lifestyle choice, that you have type 2 diabetes, particularly, because you made poor choices in your life. And that is often also put on to people with type 1 diabetes. Or the whole, 'Oh, you've got diabetes, you can't eat this, you can't do that, you should be doing this.' And so people with diabetes have a whole different set of rules from the very opinionated public and often it's not always correct, and it's not always true. And most of it's provided in kindness. But it's certainly not always received with generosity, shall we say. And I just think that that's a really big problem in itself. Because I think even within the healthcare system, there are people who don't really understand.

And because it's a chronic condition, sometimes people with diabetes are really struggling. And so sometimes, people with diabetes, like people with any condition, can be quite difficult patients. So there's not just a simple solution for everybody. It's really complex, which is why I like it.

Support

I say to all my patients, particularly people with type 1 I think it's really important, but I often say it to people with type 2 as well, that if I can help them to understand their condition, then they can go anywhere in the world, and go to any doctor, and decide if that healthcare professional or doctor knows what they're talking about, which sounds really demeaning about the healthcare profession. But I think there's a lot of people who don't understand diabetes particularly well. And when it's your condition, when it's something that I can't take away from you, but I can help you to learn to understand it. And if I can do that to the best of the patient's ability, then I think I'm doing them a good service. Because I have been known to say to people, 'This is not my disease, this is yours. This is your condition, not mine.' I can't own it for them. People have to own it, they have to accept it, and then we have to find ways to make it work for their life, within their lifestyle. And that's how I tend to approach things.

I think the biggest piece of advice I'd give people wanting to work in diabetes is don't think that you're going in there to tell people what to do, because that's not our role. Our role is to support people to manage the best they can.

When it comes to chronic care, the other thing that's so important, it doesn't matter what condition, is that people are part of a family, and whether that family is themselves and their dog … I had a man the other day who left hospital with ketones screamingly high because he had to go and feed his dog. And that was his family, so very important to him. So you're not just treating that person in that room, you're treating a whole community, or engaging with a whole community or their community.

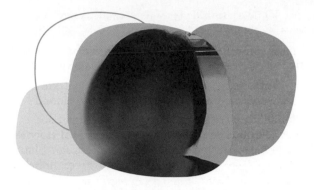

CHAPTER 12

Joey's story

Organisational challenges for looking after breast cancer patients with lymphoedema

I look after women from the very start of their breast cancer journey, from diagnosis to many, many, many years following breast cancer. Some of my patients I have followed for 30 years of their lives. So, it's been a longitudinal process. So, in general, the primary condition that I look after is lymphoedema following breast cancer. And we are now screening women for lymphoedema throughout their breast cancer journey from baseline even prior to their surgery to quite often two years, if not longer, following their breast cancer surgery.

I think that the challenges are probably threefold. There's the patient challenge, there's the organisational challenge, and then there's the challenge from my own perspective from a physio point of view. So, if you look at it from an organisational point of view, I think the problem starts in that physio or allied health, in general, isn't necessarily part of the plan when the hospital or healthcare service focus on a chronic health condition. Say, for example, most people, when you talk about funding for diabetes or funding for breast cancer, you look at the medical side of things – surgery, radiation, oncology, medical oncology and nursing. But there's little foresight put into the allied health component. So, that's the physiotherapy, the psychology, the dietitian – other things that the patient may need in their supportive care through the journey. And what happens from a public health point of view is that because of the limited funding, the resources that are available for these breast cancer patients with chronic needs, it's just not there. There's not enough hours in the day to be able to support women's demand for these services. So, that's a problem in organisational planning. And quite often some of these positions are funded just by year-to-year funding, soft funding, okay, or grant money, or things like that. And the funding may dry up in six months' time. So, do you book the patient in six months' time? Do you assume the clinic is going to continue forever? So, that's an organisation structural issue and foresight issue when it comes to public health funding. In the private, again, similar issues, in the way that patients have to pay for allied health services. It's not necessarily covered by Medicare, or their private health insurance. And some people, that presents a really big barrier. People don't necessarily want to pay. They're so focused on the medical side of things, the surgery, the radiation, oncology, and the medical oncology, that things like lymphoedema or musculoskeletal issues is lower on their priority list. And so that presents a problem.

Challenges for managing lymphoedema among women living with breast cancer

From the patient point of view, there are barriers. So, for example, in the last 10 years or so there's been a real drive to try and screen patients preoperatively for things like lymphoedema. So, trying to do baseline measurements, and follow patients up, say on a three-monthly basis, all the way up to the two-year post-axillary dissection mark, where they're most at risk of developing lymphoedema. But the problem is, and we've encountered a lot of this in the public hospital, that some patients just don't want to be monitored. They don't see that there is a problem until they develop it. They don't see the value in preventative health. They don't see the value in monitoring. But at the same time, you've got to understand it from the patient's point of view. They've got so many other medical and other nursing appointments that they've got to attend. This is just another thing to have to deal with. And they'd much rather not think about it. So, that's a bit of a challenge. But then you get the other spectrum of the scale as well. You've got people who are overly anxious about lymphoedema. People who want to be monitored every day, people who want to be monitored every week, which we just don't have the resources or the funding to be able to do. So, there is a spectrum. You've got people that don't want to attend for screening, people who just don't see the value in it. And there's the other end that people want your services all the time, almost to the extreme, where it perpetuates their fear and anxiety, which is not always needed. So, in the private side of things, the cost of accessing physiotherapy and allied health services is a big barrier, as I mentioned. In the public, it's more to do with the fact is the patient willing to come back, and are there appointments available, and are there resources available?

Challenges for looking after breast cancer patients with lymphoedema: from the physiotherapist perspective

From a health professional point of view, the major challenges in barrier is probably it's quite a niche area of physiotherapy to work in breast cancer care. And if you can imagine, most people, when they do an undergraduate or graduate degree in physiotherapy, don't necessarily fall into that specialisation pathway. Most people who graduate from physio want to do sports injuries, backs and necks; they see it as a more traditional career path or a more lucrative career path. And breast cancer care, or cancer care in general, is not probably rated as high. But that's not to say there are younger health professionals coming through who may be interested. But there are also limited numbers of positions available, and limited numbers of experienced cancer care physios who're able to mentor and tutor these up-and-coming physios who may be interested in cancer care. The other thing is people look at cancer care, or treating chronic diseases as, you know, it's not attractive, it's not an attractive specialisation career path. Where I actually think it's the reverse but I'm biased in the way I look at it. People don't see it as something that they can amend quickly. It's not like I can just give a patient a pill and everything will be resolved the next day. I think chronic illnesses, like lymphoedema, take a long time to treat. It's not necessarily a quick fix. And it takes persistence and hard work from the therapist's point of view, as well as from the patient point of view, to actually arrive at an end point that may not necessarily be a fix. It may only be management of the problem for a period of time, until they have another exacerbation, until you manage it or change your management in some other way. I think sometimes with physios and medicos they want to look after illnesses that can be fixed quickly, that they can see instant results. And that's something that chronic illnesses, we're just not able to do.

So, say you want to open a new cancer care centre, okay, I would think the majority of organisations wouldn't even have the foresight of having allied health or physio or psychologist on hand. They would devote their funding into the surgery, medical oncology, and radiation oncology, and nursing side of things.

Other hospitals do have lymphoedema services. And other hospitals do have physios available for cancer care patients. But more often than not, it's not located within the cancer care centre. It is within the physio department, so the physios will treat everything from backs and necks to breast cancer patients. But it's not co-located within the cancer care service. And it's not a blanket referral.

[My current position in cancer care] completely depends on the funding. I have been in this position for fourteen-and-a-half years, and it's still year-to-year funding. There are other health professionals in the cancer care centre that it's also on year-to-year funding as well. Some nurses here are on year-to-year funding, because they're funded by, say, Cancer Institute grant money.

There are some lymphoedema patients that I can never discharge. These patients will continue to have lymphoedema for the rest of their life. They will continue to need replacement of their compression garments and be monitored for the rest of their lives. So, I can never discharge the patients. After fourteen-and-a-half years, you start to accumulate chronic patients like these, that although they may not be seen very frequently, it certainly blocks my ability to take on new patients when there are patients I can never discharge.

I still believe that the demand is still there. Whether I'll be able to meet the demand in the future, I honestly don't know. I mean, my hours have not increased in the last fourteen-and-a-half years, so I have to say there must be a breaking point in the service where I won't be able to take on new patients.

The idea is I meet them at baseline, maybe even prior to surgery, or shortly after surgery, to inform them of their risk of lymphoedema. And some patients, it may be very low risk. Other patients, it may be quite high risk. And we figure out a plan as to how often I need to monitor them. Some patients need monitoring every three months. Other patients, I don't need to see them for six months, if not a year. So it just depends. And they are given the opportunity, and they are invited to come in to have this discussion. But what we have found is some patients just aren't interested. They really cannot give an hour in a day to come in for that conversation. They do not see it (lymphoedema) as terribly important. And it's hard to convince someone when I haven't even met them. We send them a letter in the mail to invite them. But it's up to them to give us a call.

I think COVID is a good example. So, in the last two years, some patients, understandably, have been quite fearful of COVID and have been avoiding coming to the hospital for appointments. So, there are some that I haven't seen for two years, and have just started coming out of the woodwork now, with quite significant worsening of their lymphoedema. Now, they tell me, quite often I hear this, 'oh, it's only gotten worse in the last few months'. And you look at their arm, I think this has been going on for probably the last few years rather than the last few months. And then they suddenly want an appointment now, when I've got waiting lists, obviously, for a good six weeks before they can come in.

There can be quite often a mismatch. But also, remember, what I stated from the other extreme. There are patients who have had one lymph node removed who are extremely fearful of lymphoedema. From a health professional point of view, that risk is actually very small. Now, if I have to choose, I'm going to target my resources to those who are at high risk, rather than the ones at low risk. But sometimes it's these low-risk patients that keep making appointments, and blocking my ability to see some of the high-risk patients as well.

I think it's the perception of the risk to yourself. So some people, maybe they've got lots of family support, should something happen to their arm, there are plenty of people that can help them out. Whereas other people, they may be a single parent, or a couple of kids, and they do everything, they have to work, and the perception may differ.

Yeah, it's to do with their personality. And it's not something that can be easily changed. You know, there are people who suffer from personality disorders, who have increased fear and anxiety in all aspects of life, even prior to breast cancer. And when suddenly you've got this illness that hits them, and their fear and anxiety levels rise up for everything in their life, including lymphoedema, and it's very hard to change that, because that's been an ongoing personality thing for a long time. Whereas other people, no, their attitude is it doesn't bother me, the glass half full kind of person, always see the bright side of things. They're the easiest ones to educate.

I think even if you were to train up a whole heap of physios interested in cancer, and lymphoedema care, so say we fostered a whole generation of physios interested in cancer and lymphoedema care, you've still got to have a job available for them at the end of the day. And even if every cancer care centre in Sydney had a job for a physio, you're probably only looking at, at the most, 10 jobs that are available. So, it's the supply/demand thing, okay?

So, even if you've got the funding available, there are only so many places to be able to have the experience and foster that education. Because if you don't work in cancer, if you only see one cancer patient a week, you're never going to be able to develop that experience. It's something that does require a bit of specialisation. So, if you ask me to treat a hip operation, a total hip replacement, now, I'm a physio, I should, theoretically, be able to see someone after a total hip replacement. But I can tell you, I've worked in cancer care for so many years, I'm not that confident in treating a hip, because I don't know what the recent protocols are. I don't know the latest in orthopaedic surgery. Well, similarly, to be good at what you do in cancer care, you've got to continuously see cancer and lymphoedema patients. And that's where that discord may be. There's not enough jobs available to fit in the next generation of trained physiotherapists in cancer care.

Resources and equipment needed

There is equipment that is required. For example, we use a machine called bio impedance. And that is used to measure extracellular fluid in a person's limb. And that's a fairly important tool that we use for lymphoedema assessment. The problem is it costs a lot of money. It costs about $16,000 to have such a machine.

Additionally, there may be a need for laser. And a laser costs about $6000. There's another machine called tissue dielectric constant. And these machines cost another $6000. But probably the most costly thing that adds up over time is the cost of compression garments. In particular, custom-made compression garments.

I think at the moment we could do with some extra equipment. We could do with more funding available for compression garments. Staffing-wise, we've got it about right at the moment. Unless there is another surge of patients. But we're probably still dealing with a little bit of the post-COVID, making up for lost time, from the last two years.

I think I've got the basic resources.

It is [about funding]. And I realise that with the budgets for health care, it's a little bit like robbing Peter to pay Paul. So, if you give more money to lymphoedema, you lose some money from diabetes. You know?

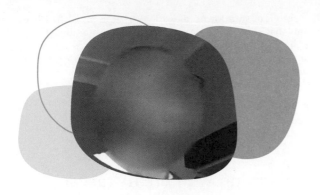

CHAPTER 12

Linda's story

Psychological challenge for women living with breast cancer

I was diagnosed in March 2020. It's always there at the back of my mind. And I suppose that's because monitoring is such a long-term project. My husband said to me the other day, 'When's your next medical appointment?' So it's always there. It's always present. I don't kind of worry about my health too much. But I'm vigilant, you know? If something went wrong, I'd be asking for assistance.

Support for going through the cancer journey for women living with breast cancer

Passage of time. I couldn't say that one thing, one element helped. It's like, I suppose, looking at cancers across the board, that there's lots of different kinds of cancers. And they're unique to each of us individually. So, I don't think there's a single thing that I could identify that helped me get through. It was just a journey. One foot in front of the other.

Impact of pandemic on breast cancer patient with new diagnosis

Most [supports] were unavailable to me. Because I was diagnosed at the commencement of the COVID outbreak, pandemic, most things were unavailable. And when it comes to family, I have a husband and that's it. I have no other family. The advice from my medical providers at that time, at the beginning of COVID, was tell everybody to stay away. You're immunocompromised. Don't come anywhere near you. So, it was an incredibly lonely journey. My husband kept going to work. And I'd been a busy, committed professional worker all of my adult life. And all of a sudden that went away. So, I had to use my own internal resources. There were no support groups available. There was no volunteerism happening at that time. There were no home visits. It was very lonely.

Challenges for women living with breast cancer

I didn't feel like a very strong person. I felt like a bit of a failure, actually. Though I've worked always in the health sector. And all of a sudden, I was the patient. But my disease was picked up on a screening mammogram. I was asymptomatic. The surgeon who examined me at diagnosis could not feel the tumours that were present. So, it was all a bit of a shock from that perspective. I found concentration very, very hard. Both from diagnosis, but especially during chemotherapy. So, my work had to go away. I couldn't concentrate to do it.

I was angry. And I expressed my anger. Not in any volatile way. But just like [why me?] So, it's me. I'm the one in four Australians who's going to be diagnosed with a cancer during their lifetime.

I talked about my feelings a lot with my husband. But that was about the limit of it. I was fortunate to have a very good communicator in my surgeon. She was great and helped me understand a lot that I thought I understood before it applied to me. But she helped a lot in those things. And also kept an eye on me, I suppose, watching out for signs of clinical depression, anxiety and other mental health aspects. It was largely me. I just had to drag myself through it. I mean, by family, there's one person. And my husband is a lovely man. He's empathetic. But he's emotionally distant, shall we say. He doesn't show his emotion easily, or much other than that. So, I could talk at him. But I didn't get much back. [The surgeon] was very helpful. Especially in the early days. Yeah.

If you'd asked me this a few months ago, I could have talked at length, I suppose, about some of the long-term sequelae from my treatment. So, I have peripheral neuropathy, for example, as an outcome from the chemotherapy treatment. And that really worried me a lot. And it did impact on some of my decisions, such as whether I would keep working or retire. And because I've been involved in health research for the last 20-odd years, the keyboard skills suddenly went. There were things like that. I've developed lymphoedema. So, I'm living with and coping with that. There was a lot of mental health stuff. I thought that the depression had been dealt with, but it wasn't. I needed more time. And I was very reluctant to take antidepressants. So, I guess I just had to nurse myself through that and wait for the cloud to lift a bit. And the cloud comes back every so often. It doesn't take much that the wheels fall off. And I can feel pretty blue on some days.

Cabin fever. Being shut in. Not having, I guess, the liberty, because of shutdowns and things, that even if I had been well, to go out and do things or join the world. So, there was that sort of two-year hiatus of doing nothing. Doing nothing – trying to get better. And at the same time, having clinicians tell me 'Go for a walk. Do exercise.' I'm going, 'I can't do exercise. I can't go out.' You know? What am I going to do? So, I felt like some of the clinicians were experiencing a world different to the one that I was in. But even though they were well and truly aware of some of the social limitations, it was really unhelpful to keep hearing, 'Oh, you know, fix everything by going for a walk.' That didn't work for me.

[Rating the challenges on a scale from one to ten] Ten. Eleven, if I could put it on that scale. I was very challenged. Yeah.

Limited resources for supporting women living with breast cancer

There was very, very little available in terms of support. The things that I knew of, as supportive, either therapies or interventions or groups were totally unavailable because of their volunteerism or other barriers to a public hospital having those things run. So, the wig library didn't run. Look Good, Feel Better didn't run. There were no support groups that I could find, where you could just even have a chat with somebody. The oncology liaison nurse at the hospital where I was treated was welcoming. But I think she was so overloaded that I never felt that I could just phone up and go 'Ah. I'm having a bad day. I feel terrible.' I'm sure that if I had done that, that she would have met that as well as her current resources allowed. But I knew that her resources were very thin.

I would also put a caveat on that and say because my experience was during COVID, it may be totally different now. Or with [inaudible] beforehand, it was just that window. I was unfortunate.

But it was also very difficult to source any supportive therapies, massage, acupuncture, diet, exercise. Those things kind of went away as well. Yeah.

I did [try to find a support group]. And it wasn't through the hospital where I was treated. It was through my own initiative. But I found it. And I joined a dragon boat crew. And dragon boating has been found to be particularly helpful for women living with upper limb lymphoedema. And that was my main impetus, I suppose, to join. But they're a bunch of women like me. Some of their experiences of breast cancer were 30 years ago. And some of them were last week. So, it's a whole lot of women with breast cancer who happen to paddle in a boat together. So, that's been helpful. [It has been for] a year. I go to training twice a week. And paddle on Pittwater. And it's nice.

I would love it if the government could look at the German model where women who've been treated for breast cancer go off to residential camp for a couple of weeks. Where there's all sorts of assistance where they are linking them back into community-based services. But for that initial period, it's kind of like being able to have a big verbal dump. And maybe explore the things that are worrying them or their experiences. I would have loved to have had something like that. Talking to women who maybe had the same kinds of treatment. And how they coped with the inevitable side effects. And the downsides of treatment.

[Support or resources are] very difficult to navigate. I'm being treated [for lymphoedema] through a public teaching hospital. And when it comes to support garments and things, support sleeves and stuff, I bought my first one at considerable expense. And if you need to have them made, tailormade effectively, they're really expensive. And I'm six foot tall. And kind of, you know, on the large end of female physiognomy. So, I need to have them made. And it's super expensive. Now, there is a support program. But I found out about that through one of my paddling colleagues who knew about this support service. Now, I put an application to be considered for financial support for lymphoedema garments in July. I'm still waiting. So, I'm without a garment. I don't know what the lymphoedema is doing. Those things have been a bit worrying. And they're a bit concerning.

It's quite a gap between appointments. And then, having said that, I think that if you are in dire need, individuals are very willing to shift heaven and hell to try and do their best. But you know, there's finite resources. So, once you're in the system, it's much easier to navigate. But it's that entry into the system. That's the hard bit.

Challenges of medical follow-up for women living with breast cancer

I would really like to think that when I went to see my medical oncologist that he had a little bit more time and could be a bit more relaxed. It's like a factory, you know? One person in. One person out. And I mean, what's going on in that guy's head? Dealing with a whole lot of us who – I guess that the people that he sees cover such a broad spectrum. And if he's giving really bad news to somebody, and then I walk in next saying, 'Oh, you know, this peripheral neuropathy is really getting me down.' He's going 'Yeah, but you're going to live, you know? The person in front of you and the person behind you, they're stage 4 people. They're going to die quickly, and not very well.'

The other thing is that you naively believe that the appointment you've been given says you're going to see the medical oncologist. And you get the medical oncologist's registrar. And I understand the need for education and for registrars to be exposed. But sometimes it would feel, ugh, you know? I'd have to go through my whole history with the registrar. And say, this doesn't work for me. And have them sort of do a little bit of tea potting and say, 'Well, it works for everybody else.' Well, that's nice. But you know, I'm not everybody else. And people will, again, because big teaching hospital, the radiation oncologist I saw once for five minutes. And every other time I went through treatment or follow-up, it was a registrar. So, 25 treatments over six-odd weeks, I didn't see that person once. Sometimes I felt that the registrar's knowledge, especially when you knew that it was a new intake, and these people were fresh out of the box. Anything that I asked them, they'd have to go back to the medical oncologist and check with anyway. And so, I'm thinking I could have asked that question directly. And the medical oncologist could say, yes or no, or it's like this. And I would have been quite satisfied. But my confidence was lower in those registrars.

[How often I see the medical oncologist is] still being worked out. Because I had a bit of a bumpy ride with the hormone therapy. Initially I was seeing somebody from medical oncology more often. But it's been stretched out now to six months. And I believe probably the next time I go it might be stretched out to 12 months. But having said that, because I'm not tolerating that drug therapy, I need to be followed up a little more cautiously for things like bone scans, DEXA scan, just to see that I haven't got any hot spots breaking out. So I have to push for that. But there's no kind of instant recall, 'Oh yeah! She's not having that drug therapy. Therefore, she's at higher risk of recurrence.' I wouldn't like to be a shy shrinking violet and not push for it. Or I suppose I have a little bit better understanding of the disease process and even hospital processes than other women who may not have had the working environment that I've had.

Challenge of psychological and informational support for women living with breast cancer

One of the key information support aspects that I was really disappointed by was before commencing chemotherapy, my husband and I went along for what they called an information session. And in that session, which was with a nurse, we were given information about the likely side effects from chemotherapy. And I found through experience that the proposed side effects were always given at the positive end of the spectrum and didn't cover down to the negative end. And that's what I needed to know. And so, when you experience these things, and you go, 'Hang on. The nurse said this could be a transient symptom. Or only 3% of the population of women who undergo this therapy experience this symptom.' Well, I'm one of them, you know? What do you do? And the severity, and I suppose the length of the treatment as well as the timing of courses. So, my courses were typically three weeks apart. So, you have this immediate clunk of ill health. You slowly climb out of it, and then it's time for the next treatment. So, it was this incessant, you know? It's not even Napoleon's hat. There was no confidence intervals. I've worked with 95% confidence intervals all my life.

I think [psychological support] has to come through communication. And generally, I didn't feel particularly comfortable expressing that I felt that I may have been depressed. It was only my surgeon who would say, 'You're looking terrible, you know? I think you're depressed. What do you think?' Yeah. I agree. So, I think the communication skills of some of the clinicians I saw were not great. They either didn't have the time – probably I would reckon time – to be able to go, 'Oh, crikey, this lady needs to be referred to a psychologist or other mental health interventionist to have a look at what's going on.' And basically for me, it was the talking cure that once I could blah! get it out, that was it. And I saw both private- and public-sector psychologists. And none of those people actually worked with me to steer a course out of depression. And partly that could have been down to me because I declined antidepressants every time they were offered. I would have liked to have thought there were other options other than drug therapy for treating depression. But none were offered.

[The psychologists] were helpful in as much as they gave me a venue to vent, to explain the things that were worrying me. That was positive. The only nurses I saw were in the chemotherapy unit. And they're like any other group of professionals; there are good communicators, there are less good communicators.

I really appreciated nurses not coming with an assumption of, you know, this is a 60-something woman who's a bit stupid. And she won't know, or she won't understand or whatever. And that's not me. You know? I might have grey hair, but I have an active and real need to know. Some nurses got that completely and some didn't. I wouldn't know. I mean, one instance I can clearly remember was that my chemo was running one day. And a nurse came past and she wasn't treating me but she came and looked at the bag and went, 'How long has this been running?' And I told her. And she said, 'I think they've put the wrong drug up on you.' And I went, 'Oh. Let's just stop it running, shall we?' And she said, 'Yeah, I think so.' So, she went off and got the pharmacist and other nurses. And it turned out that the drug that had been put up for me was the correct drug. But it was the wrong dosage. So then there's all these people coming around and saying, 'Don't panic. We'll just titrate the dosage. But it may mean that you got more of the drug more quickly than we would have anticipated.' And they went off and did their calculations. And said, 'It's okay. We'll recalibrate. We'll put a new bag up and it won't kill you.' Oh, that's good. It was a bit scary. But the nurse who'd been responsible for putting it up – and I tried to make light of it almost with him. And I didn't want him to feel like he was going to be victimised or whatever. We all make mistakes. And it was late in the day. God knows what he'd been through that day. But in his presence, I did thank the nurse who'd been vigilant and just passing, and just go, 'That's the wrong size bag for what you are having.' And, 'Thank you for speaking up on my behalf.' And this guy was kind of sullen and head down. And after that, it sort of tainted our relationship. That I did notice it whenever I came into the unit after that, he was kind of a bit absent.

And I can understand that. I'm sure his world was rocked because he'd made a mistake.

And then another time when it was really cold weather. And you know, I'm just a person for whom cold weather, it makes me cough. But then I walked into the unit and I coughed during COVID. Not a good thing. Don't ever walk into a chemo unit and cough. And they put me in a separate room. And I felt victimised. I tried to explain. But I was pretty sure that I didn't have an infection. It was just a reaction to the cold air. But I was shuffled out. And I had to go across campus to go and get a COVID test. And it meant that that treatment had to be rescheduled. And it was just another layer.

I'm at pains to say to people that my experience was during COVID. And I think in normal health circumstances, it may not be as tricky to navigate. I think that given the strange world we were in when I was diagnosed and treated, that I have no complaints about any of the health care that I received. But people were exploring about having to invent new ways of doing things, applying protocols that hadn't been applied before. I think everybody was exemplary, yeah. I'm glad that I was in Australia when I was diagnosed. I was frightened, you know? Don't underestimate how fearful people can be with their treatment.